THE QUIET MIND
Techniques For Transforming Stress

1-800-847-8100
Songs of worship

Techniques For Transforming Stress

THE QUIET MIND

EDITED BY
JOHN HARVEY, Ph.D.

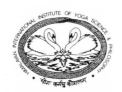

The Himalayan International Institute
of Yoga Science and Philosophy of the U.S.A.
Honesdale, Pennsylvania

© 1988 Himalayan International Institute
of Yoga Science and Philosophy of the U.S.A.
RR 1, Box 400
Honesdale, Pennsylvania 18431

Second Printing 1993

Library of Congress Cataloging in Publication Data:

The Quiet mind: techniques for transforming stress / edited by
    John R. Harvey.
        p.   cm.
    Bibliography: p.
    ISBN 0-89389-096-0
    1. Stress (Psychology)—Prevention. 2. Relaxation. 3. Meditation.
I. Harvey, John R., 1945-
RC455.4.S87Q53 1988
613.7′9—dc19
                                        88-12055
                                             CIP

Quiet minds cannot be perplexed or frightened, but go on in fortune or misfortune at their own private pace, like a clock in a thunderstorm.

—Robert Louis Stevenson

Contents

Section II. A New Understanding of Stress

Acknowledgments

The most essential support for the completion of this book came from Swami Rama. His inspired example, tireless teaching, and practical encouragement made this book possible. I hope that the ideas, guidance, and knowledge put forth in this book are a true expression of his work.

Grateful acknowledgment must go as well to Kay Gendron, Ph.D., whose patient and creative editing were a great help in bringing this book to completion. The editorial suggestions of Phil Nuernberger, Ph.D. were also very helpful during the final editing.

Foreword

by Swami Rama

The editor of this book, Dr. John Harvey, has done a great service to the reader by compiling together in one book so much useful material on stress, stress management, and the diverse approaches one can utilize to move beyond stress to self management and self-transformation.

A well-respected psychologist and teacher, Dr. Harvey has also been a faculty member of the Himalayan Institute for many years, and has made many contributions to its programs. His work in editing this book and authoring a number of its chapters is also a great service and contribution to the work of the Institute. His understanding of both Eastern and Western approaches to psychology and self-development is evident throughout. I know that through this book many individuals will become interested and challenged to begin or to intensify the process of taking responsibility for their physical health, emotional well-being, and spiritual and personal development.

When an individual learns to appreciate the methods of stress transformation, he experiences remarkable changes in his internal states and he becomes aware of those dimensions of life which are not ordinarily known. He experiences these dimensions of life consciously and they help him to expand his consciousness. He can then fathom those deeper levels of life that are fulfilling and unfolding.

The deeper one goes, the more one also attains the higher dimensions of the summit. The mind becomes one-pointed, inward, and free from external stimuli and pain. Such a mind becomes a great tool for him to use to know the subtleties of life.

It is essential to have a one-pointed and penetrating mind to do research in the interior world, for nothing external helps us, and the only available tool is the mind. I don't know of any therapy that affects one perfectly without first having an even mind, and to develop an even mind, a serene breathing pattern and a well-nourished body are equally essential. Therefore the therapy should involve all levels—the physical body, the breath (the energy level), and the mental level. When the body, breath, and mind are perfectly coordinated, then human awareness expands. This expansion helps one to treat and help others.

Ordinarily, a common man is agitated by emotional outbursts because he has not learned to channel his energy physically, to breathe serenely, or to think in a positive way. The power of positive thinking is immense and establishing serene breath helps the nervous system to remain a proper channel to allow the energy to flow and to establish coordination in the limbs.

To be free from one specific emotional problem is not real learning, because again another emotion can disturb the emotional body. The emotional body is like a fish in the water of our inner lake. If our thinking and emotions are not organized, then that emotional body is consciously disturbed and those disturbances can be termed and classified in many ways. It is healthy to follow the whole process of treating a patient on all levels—body, breath, and mind.

If the patient is led to treat himself it is also a great solace for the therapist to know that his method works effectively, instead of lingering slowly and trying to weave yarns together by pulling one thread at a time, for the fabric of the inner life is intricately and artistically woven by nature. To understand all this, a definite methodology and technology is applied: nourishing diet, exercise according to one's comfortable capacity, and breath techniques which are helpful, such as deep diaphragmatic breathing, alternate breathing, and retention according to one's capacity. It is important to know that understanding the breath is essential. Learning how to think positively also has a great value in life. This approach will help the aspirant to understand the origins of the conflicts created by the mind and projected through the nervous system and body. Conflict within and without play prime roles in human life. Experiencing less conflict will free the human mind from stress.

Freedom from stress is a necessity for modern man. However, learning not to allow oneself to live in stress is a holistic approach that can be practiced by everyone—men, women, and children. Through this process of gaining freedom from stress and increasing individual self-awareness and self-responsibility, our present society itself will be transformed.

All human beings face challenges and difficulties in dealing with the external world. There will always be unfortunate events to face and conflicts to resolve. But it is important for human beings to become aware of one thing—that they have within them a vast untapped capacity that is far more powerful than these external means and crutches. And, more importantly, that this potential can be understood, experienced, and realized, that human beings can definitely develop themselves far beyond their present understanding—to experience a state of stressless balance and harmony—physically, mentally, and on all levels. When this occurs, human beings become increasingly creative, dynamic, and peaceful. This is not merely an idealistic statement that applies only to some particularly fortunate individuals, but to all who are willing to begin the process of increasing their self-awareness and self-control. For those who undertake this process there are clear and impressive rewards.

I know that the Board of Directors of the Himalayan Institute will join me in thanking Dr. John Harvey for his many hours of tireless and selfless service on this and many other projects. We share our gratitude as well with his wife, Dawn Harvey, who has been supportive of him in this creative venture.

—Swami Rama

Stress: An Introduction

Stress is an exciting problem. It is a problem because the effects of stress are very destructive to health, productivity, and the expression of human potential. It is exciting because the same approaches and techniques that we utilize to reduce stress also have the potential to become a vehicle for improving physical health, enhancing mental skills, and facilitating self-expression. These methods of stress management can even become the foundation of a systematic program of self-development. It is, however, the problematic and negative aspects of stress that have drawn the most attention and concern. Therefore, before we consider the more exciting implications of stress management let us explore the problematic aspects in greater detail.

The term *stress* in this "problem" sense has become quite common in everyday speech and often enters into most people's thinking about their own lives. Almost everyone admits that they are experiencing some degree of stress and that stress is certainly a problem for modern society. Yet most of us are not aware of the full depth and breadth of the stress problem. Some facts and figures from a recent *Time* magazine article illustrate the gravity of the situation.[1]

-Two thirds of the office visits to family doctors are prompted by stress-related symptoms.

-Stress-related absenteeism, company medical expenses, and lost productivity may cost between $50-75 billion a year.

-Stress is now known to be a major contributor, either directly or indirectly, to six of the leading causes of death in the U.S., namely, coronary heart disease, cancer, lung ailments, accidental injuries, cirrhosis of the liver and suicide.

-The three best selling prescription medications in the country, (Valium, Inderal and Tagamet) treat problems either caused or aggravated by stress, namely, anxiety, hypertension, and ulcers.

Further definition of the seriousness of the stress problem is provided by noted cardiologist Robert Eliot in his book, *Is It Worth Dying For?* He states categorically that, "Stress may be the greatest single contributor to illness in the industrialized world."[2] Along these lines stress is considered to affect the onset, treatment, or recovery from such major illnesses as cardiovascular disease, cancer, diabetes mellitus, tuberculosis, rheumatoid arthritis, hypertension, ulcers, neuromuscular pain conditions, allergies, common colds and pre-menstrual tension. But physical illness is not the only domain where stress wreaks havoc; emotional health and mental functions such as memory, concentration, and creativity are also impaired. Behavioral efficiency, interpersonal relationships, and personal productivity are also limited by stress. In this light, it is evident that stress is a significant problem.

In the face of this evidence it is clear that the problem of stress must be addressed on all levels. Comprehensive stress management and approaches to behavioral health problems can be implemented in the workplace in order to hold down health care costs, boost productivity, and increase morale. And, in fact, many corporations are currently offering programs in stress reduction, smoking cessation, and weight control, and some are devoting considerable resources to the development of comprehensive and coordinated programs for positive lifestyle change.[3] At the same time, the nation's health care industry needs to reduce stress-related illness to try and hold skyrocketing health care costs in check. Action on this front is reflected in the proliferation of hospital-based "Wellness" programs. But most importantly, each individual can benefit tremendously by taking responsibility for managing stress in his or her own life.

If such corporate and community-wide programs are put into effect, if a general consciousness develops regarding the importance of stress management, and if, as a result, many individuals begin to consistently practice management in their daily lives, then the door is opened upon the *exciting* and dynamic aspects of stress management. The ability to regulate all of the inner systems is the essence of stress management. This means learning to gracefully control mind, muscles, nervous system, and endocrine system. We can use these inner control skills to reduce the excessive and destructive activation associated with stress. Yet these same skills provide us with an opportunity to develop our fullest potential.

The inner skills of stress management serve as a foundation for self development. A parallel may be seen with the great traditions of self-transformation, such as Yoga, Sufism, and Zen Buddhism. In each of these traditions, an initial and basic step on the journey of self-transformation is learning to be aware of, and to regulate the various dimensions of body, mind, and emotions. Once these basic skills are mastered, a person has begun to awaken and the true process of self-transformation may begin. In the same vein, a person who practices stress management is changed. He becomes more of an *insider,* more aware of his inner potential, and better able to creatively improve himself at all levels. The techniques of stress management are like a coin: on one side the inscription is "stress management," and we use the skills to react to a crucial and destructive problem. But if we turn the coin over, the inscription reads "self-transformation," and we have begun an exciting journey.

In this transformational sense, we can use such techniques as relaxation, concentration, mastery of perception and regulation of our thought patterns to enhance our creativity, decisiveness, and intuition. We can understand how to use exercise and diet to positively affect and improve the mind/body complex. But more importantly, as we establish a process of inner awareness and regulation we begin to understand the subtle origins of stress and illness in our attitudes, beliefs, and in our philosophy of life. We come to see the manner in which we can transform ourselves at these most crucial levels of being. We begin to sense how our attitudes and beliefs, our improved outlook on life, and even our developing spiritual understanding create an inner environment that allows for the realization of our fullest potentials.

Stress management techniques are not inert, neutral, mechanical tools. They are powerful and dynamic instruments—they begin processes of change. The person who practices stress management consistently and thoroughly is irrevocably changed. This change has tremendous positive potential and clearly represents the exciting aspect of stress. We are challenged by stress to take responsibility for our mind, body, and spirit. Once we have assumed this responsibility we have created an opportunity for self-directed personal growth.

This book is compiled with both aspects of stress in mind. We must understand the problem of stress and develop practical methods for dealing with it. This, indeed, is the focus of the first section of this anthology. Then we may begin to explore the interface between the reactive, problem-reducing nature of stress management and the potential for self-transformation. This is done in the second section by enhancing our understanding of stress and by probing into the more subtle aspects of stress causation and stress management. In this section we also are presented with a framework for understanding mind-body-spirit interactions that allow us to better appreciate the dynamic aspects of stress management.

The third and last section of the book focuses more directly on the self-transformational aspects of stress management. Here the techniques, strategies, and understandings of yoga are presented not only as a means for restoring physical and emotional harmony or for gaining inner awareness, but also as methods for self-development and self-transformation.

The goal of this book is that the reader will gain a precise understanding of the nature of stress, and that he or she will also gain the tools necessary to effectively reduce stress and thereby avoid unnecessary illness and suffering. At the same time, the reader may become increasingly aware of how these stress management techniques can enhance performance. Ultimately, the reader may come to feel the profound positive potential of this inner technology and to see how it can be used to effect a transformation on all levels of his or her being. As this transformation occurs the door is opened for the realization of each individual's fullest potential.

SECTION I.

Practical Approaches to Stress Management

CHAPTER 1

An Overview of Stress and Stress Management

John R. Harvey, Ph.D.

A friend came into my office recently looking very concerned. He related how his great grandfather, a hearty and robust immigrant from Europe, had enjoyed good health until he suffered a heart attack at the age of 78. His grandfather, a self-made man, who started and ran his own business, had his heart attack at age 68. His father, a hard-driving professional, was only 58 when he was stricken with a fatal heart attack. My friend looked down, let out a long sigh and in a resigned tone said, "I suppose I won't make it past 48." After some moments of silence his energy returned, he looked up and asked, "Why is this happening? Why are the men in my family dying earlier and earlier?" Again he fell into silence and then suddenly with a note of determination, he asked me, "Is there something I can do to prevent this from happening to me?"

I've often reflected on this meeting with my friend. For him the questions were timely. He was in a crisis, but ready to make changes in his life. And he has made them and is now in excellent health. But I find that similar questions are raised by many others. They look at the progress of their own families through the generations, moving ahead financially, achieving more material success, and yet the success does not seem to come alone. With each successive generation success is increasingly accompanied by the specter of illness and early death. It is quite natural to wonder, what is the cause of this problem and if anything can be done about it.

Fortunately there are answers to both of these questions. Stress is the major cause of these health problems. Stress is a great killer and its impact has increased with each generation as the pace of society has speeded up and become more complex. And there is something that can be done about it. We can learn to manage stress. But these answers actually raise a lot more questions. What is stress? How does it wreak such havoc on our health? How can it be prevented? What can we do to avoid it? Let us begin to answer these questions by probing into the nature of the stress response.

While stress itself has probably existed for centuries, the concept and the label are relatively modern. The use of the term "stress" in reference to humans stems from the work of the eminent researcher Hans Selye, who in the 1930s discovered a generalized internal response of living organisms to environmental challenges. When confronted with such demands as exposure to chemicals, extreme temperatures, and loud noises, organisms showed a dramatic and comprehensive pattern of internal mobilization, a stress response, to prepare them to deal with this threat. In scientific terms, Selye described stress as "the non-specific response of the body to any demand."[1]

Selye's discovery of the stress response was actually somewhat indirect. While doing research on the effects of sex hormones, he injected various ovarian and placental extracts into laboratory rats and noticed three dramatic effects. The rats exposed to these extracts showed an enlargement of the outer layer of the adrenal cortex, a shrinking of the thymus, and the appearance of deep, bleeding ulcers in the lining of the stomach. He noted that the more of the hormone he injected, the more dramatic this response triad was. He was thrilled, and was convinced that he was on the path to identifying a very important and significant sex hormone. However, his happiness turned to great disappointment when subsequent research showed that the same effect occurred if any extract or other chemical was injected.

It is to Selye's great credit that, despite his deep disappointment, he was able to view his findings creatively from another perspective. He describes this process as follows: "Eventually I decided that, of course, the only reasonable thing to do was to pull myself together, admit my defeat, and return to some of the more orthodox endocrinologic problems that had occupied my attention before I was sidetracked into this regrettable enterprise. After all, I was young and much of the road still lay ahead. Yet, somehow I could not forget my triad, nor could I get hold of myself sufficiently to do anything else in the laboratory for several days."[2]

Selye goes on to describe a period of contemplation of his data that ultimately became very important for his career and for the field of stress. He began to realize that his triad represented a generalized response of the organism to an external demand, in this case a foreign substance. He later found that a wide variety of chemicals as well as such environmental factors as cold, heat, X-rays, mechanical trauma, pain, and forced exercise would also induce this response. He felt that the response represented the mobilization of the animal's resources to deal with a threat. Accordingly, he named the response the "Alarm triad," and with this the study of the stress syndrome had begun.

Selye's continuing research revealed that this stress response was even more complex than he had initially imagined, and that it seemed to change and evolve over time. For example, he found that the activation of what he called an alarm reaction was followed by a state of resistance or adaptation wherein the animal seemed to adjust to the threat or demand. The harmful effects of the alarm response seemed to fade away. But then came a third stage, in which the symptoms returned and the organism showed excessive wear and tear. The animal seemed to suffer from premature aging and was at risk for sickness and death. Selye named this phase the "stage of exhaustion."

Selye labeled the combination of these three stages the "General Adaptation Syndrome," or G.A.S. This model of the G.A.S. has been the basis for considerable further research into stress and for an understanding of the stress response in humans. Selye believed that if stress responding was excessive and continued over sufficient time, then the stress diseases or the diseases of adaptation will set in. He also theorized that each person has a certain store of adaptive energy. If this store is used up through excessive stress responding, then accelerated wear and tear occur, somewhat like premature aging, and eventually breakdowns in the body will also occur.

The Stress Response

Subsequently, the exact unfolding of the stress response in humans has been considered and researched in great detail. Dr. Mary Asterita has drawn upon this research and presents the following schema for understanding the human stress response in her book, *The Physiology of Stress*.[3]

To begin with, Asterita states that the stress response starts with activity in the brain. We respond to some event, which may be either something happening in the environment, or something internal such as a thought, memory, or feeling. We process this event mentally and if a perception of a threat registers, a part of the brain known as the limbic system is activated. This limbic system, deep within the brain, is an archaic anatomical structure that humans share with all other vertebrates. Structurally unchanged in

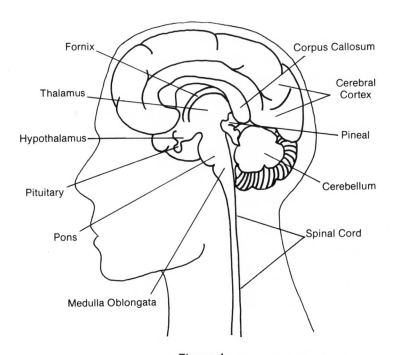

Figure 1
Central Nervous System: The Brain and Spinal Cord
Source: Nuernberger: *Freedom from Stress: A Holistic Approach*

humankind over the centuries, it is known to govern emotional responses and motivational states, and to organize the accompanying physiological arousal. Within the limbic system a small gland known as the hypothalamus (Figure 1) receives the encoded signal of an emotional reaction and begins the process of activating the initial physiological aspects of the stress response.

Before we trace the manner in which this response unfolds, it is important to keep in mind that our brain processes things in a complex, interactive manner. There are patterns in the brain that determine what will arouse our attention and begin the appraisal of threat. There is also a drawing on the memory of past experiences or learning that determines the degree and extent of the appraisal of threat. Accordingly, this initial appraisal stage very much involves our mental habits and can be expected to be unique to each person.

Once the thinking and sensing parts of our brain have determined that some threat is present and that there may be some need to take action, then the hypothalamus activates the autonomic nervous system (ANS). The ANS controls and regulates basic, inner body processes such as heart rate, respiration, blood pressure, hormonal balance, metabolism, and the functioning of the reproductive system. The ANS controls all the inner aspects of the body in a marvelously coordinated fashion so that we have more energy and a greater intensity of inner activity to deal with external demands. An illustration of the ANS is provided in Figures 2 and 3.

The activation that occurs as a response to threat is accomplished through one branch of the ANS, known as the sympathetic branch because in a sense it is in sympathy with or supportive of activation. The sympathetic aspect of the stress response occurs quickly and brings on an increase in heart rate, heart metabolism, blood pressure, sweat production, brain activity, muscle strength, and basal metabolism. Blood sugar levels rise as the liver effects an enhanced release of glucose. Simultaneously there is a decrease in blood flow to the periphery of the body, producing the effect of cold, clammy hands. There is also a decrease in blood flow to the digestive tract and a decrease in peristaltic activity.

It is less important to remember all of these specific effects than it is to keep in mind the idea of an immediate and total inner mobilization of the body through the action of the sympathetic branch of the ANS. This sudden and massive activation in our body is what we feel when we have a near miss with another car on the freeway or before we step to the podium to give a talk. We feel a pounding heart, a queasy stomach, shaky knees, increased sweating, cold, clammy hands, a dry mouth, and perhaps a cracking voice. This immediate activation of the sympathetic nervous system prepares us totally for action and is known as the "fight or flight" response. It is this response that we typically associate with stress.

But it is important to point out that there is another branch of the ANS known as the parasympathetic. Its function is more or less opposite and complementary to the sympathetic branch. It is concerned with internal housekeeping, relaxation, and restoration of the body. Ideally the sympathetic and parasympathetic branches work in a balanced and complementary fashion, so that activation and relaxation alternate, and so that the activation of the ANS is appropriately tuned to the activity at hand: one level for quiet work, another for dealing with an emergency, another for eating, another for loving, and so on. Table 1 provides an overview of the bodily functions affected by the ANS.

Table 1
Effects of ANS Stimulation

Organ or Function	Sympathetic Branch	Parasympathetic Branch
Heart	increased rate	decreased rate
	increased force of contraction	decreased force of contraction
Stomach	decreased peristalsis	increased peristalsis
Blood pressure	increased	decreased
Bronchi (lungs)	dilated	constricted
Sweat glands	copious sweating	none
Liver	glucose released	slight glycogen synthesis
Pupils (eyes)	dilated	constricted
Metabolism	increased	none
Adrenal hormone secretion	increased	none
Peripheral vasoconstriction	increased	none
Mental activity	increased	none
Biloerector muscles	excited	none
Skeletal muscles	increased strength	none
Kidneys	decreased output	none

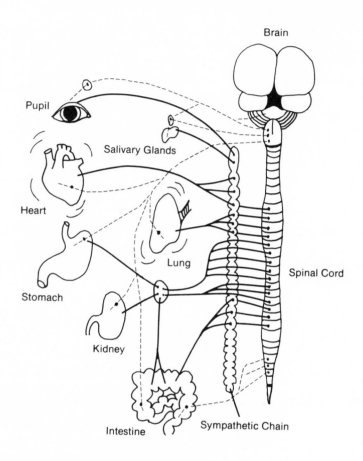

Increased Sympathetic Activity ————————

Decreased Parasympathetic Activity _ _ _ _ _ _ _ _ _ _

Figure 2
Sympathetic System Dominant
Source: Nuernberger: *Freedom from Stress: A Holistic Approach*

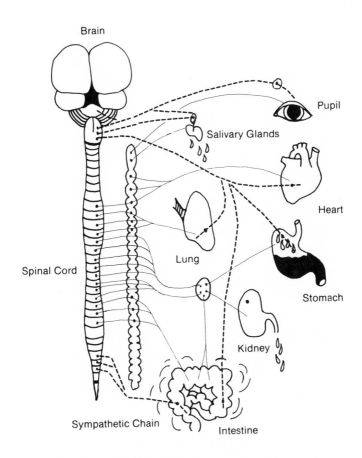

Decreased Sympathetic Activity _____
Increased Parasympathetic Activity -------------

Figure 3
Parasympathetic System Dominant

Source: Nuernberger: *Freedom from Stress: A Holistic Approach*

Too much sympathetic activity can create stress, but there can also be too much parasympathetic response if the body slows down and relaxes too much. Significant decreases in heart rate and blood pressure can produce fainting or even life-threatening cardiac arrhythmias. Whereas sympathetic branch activation is often initiated by the appraisal of a threat, excessive parasympathetic response is often set off by the perception of a total loss of control. This is an equally significant form of stress. However, at this time much more is known about the physiology of the fight or flight response and we will consider that in greater detail.

A second phase of the fight or flight response involves the release of stress hormones into the bloodstream. This second phase intensifies and maintains the impact of the initial autonomic response. This phase is triggered by the sympathetic nervous system's stimulation of the core of the adrenal gland. This gland, situated atop the kidneys, releases potent stress hormones, known as catecholamines, into the bloodstream.

Two of these hormones, epinephrine and norepinephrine, are particularly important in this second phase of the stress response; they act to intensify the stress response and maintain it through time. Epinephrine acts to increase blood sugar, boost metabolism, increase the heart rate, and stimulate the central nervous system. Norepinephrine also increases the heart rate, but acts to increase bronchodilation, blood pressure, and vasoconstriction as well. Together, these powerful hormones lead to an even more thorough mobilization of the body. In terms of physiological arousal, the body is now exquisitely prepared either for fight or flight.

Then a third phase follows, in which the body acts to strengthen and maintain the stress response across time. A chain reaction occurs in which the hypothalamus releases a hormone that stimulates part of the pituitary gland to produce another hormone. This new hormone, in turn, stimulates the outer layer of the adrenal gland to produce another important stress hormone known as cortisol. Cortisol bolsters the stress response by increasing protein mobilization, fat mobilization, and the formation of glucose. Obviously these changes draw on the body's available resources in order to provide extra energy to maintain the stress response. The release of cortisol, while beneficial in the immediate stress response, does however, depress the effectiveness of the immune system.

The role of cortisol illustrates clearly an important issue in the stress response. There is nothing necessarily wrong with our producing cortisol; it is a natural and adaptive response that provides the energy we need to deal with an external demand. But there is a trade-off: if we mobilize for the short term, the body redirects its adaptive energy to that mobilization. Long-term concerns such as the repair and regeneration of the body and the maintenance of the immune system are then simply put at a lower priority. This is fine if we deal with a demand and then let go. But if we maintain this intense activation over time, it is obvious that we are decreasing the body's ability to take care of itself and are thereby inviting disease.

Overview of the Fight Or Flight Response

Phase 1. ANS Sympathetic Activation (Instant Activation)

Action
1. Perception of internal or external event
2. Cortical appraisal of threat
3. Activation of limbic system
4. Hypothalamus activates ANS

Effects
Heart rate increases, blood pressure rises, glucose is released, metabolism rises, mental activity increases, skeletal muscles are strengthened, vasoconstriction increases, stomach motility decreases.

Result
Body instantly activated and ready to take action.

Phase 2. Hormones Released from Adrenal Medulla (Full Mobilization)

Action

1. ANS sympathetic stimulation acts to release hormones from adrenal medulla.
2. Catecholamines, especially epinephrine and norepinephrine, are released into bloodstream.

Effects

Epinephrine increases blood sugar, metabolism, heart rate and activation of CNS. Norepinephrine increases heart rate, bronchodilation, blood pressure, and peripheral vasoconstriction.

Result

Body is now fully mobilized either to fight or flee.

Phase 3. Stress Hormone Release from Adrenal Cortex (Long-Term Mobilization)

Action

1. Hypothalamus releases a hormone that stimulates anterior pituitary.
2. Pituitary gland releases a hormone that stimulates adrenal cortex.
3. Adrenal cortex releases cortisol into bloodstream.

Effects

Cortisol increases protein mobilization, fat mobilization, and blood sugar levels, and decreases inflammation and immune system activity.

Result

Body is now prepared to maintain a high level of activation over a long period of time.

In summary, the three stages described represent the major physiological activity of the fight or flight response. There are, however, additional physiological changes that should be mentioned at least briefly to give some idea of the full complexity of the stress response. For example, the impact of the stress response on the endocrine glands may alter the regulation of circadian rhythms in the body. The release of endogenous opiates may act to increase pain resistance and affect behavior and learning. In males, the production of testosterone by the testes is suppressed. In females, the monthly cycle of hormone production can alter, and consequently the menstrual cycle may be affected. Furthermore, in both sexes the metabolism of vitamins, minerals, and other nutrients may be affected by the stress response.

This activation response is complex and affects all aspects of our physiology. Certain physiological functions—such as blood pressure, heart rate, ANS change, and the secretion of stress hormones—occur in most people in a somewhat similar fashion. But, as Asterita points out, "When the more chronic neuroendocrine phase of the stress response occurs, it occurs with a greater amount of variability. Many of the endocrine components may or may not be stimulated, but when stimulated it is with varying degrees of intensity."[4] Thus, the types of demands we are exposed to, the nature of our cognitive interpretation, the intensity and duration of our stress response, and our genetic inheritance all interact to determine the impact and effect that stress has on us.

The Effects of Stress

The effects of stress are quite dramatic. Selye's work and considerable other research provide a good overview of these effects. Nowhere has the impact of stress been better documented than in research on heart disease, a health problem identified as having a significant component of stress causation. The effects of the stress chemicals secreted by the adrenal gland are of particular importance in contributing to heart disease. Epinephrine acts to elevate blood pressure, which in itself is a health risk. This silent killer takes a number of years to wreak its havoc, but untreated, elevated blood pressure sooner or later leads to some organ failure. High blood pressure damages and narrows the large arteries that bring blood and the necessary nutrients and oxygen to all the tissues in the body.

A common organ system breakdown for high blood pressure is kidney failure, which occurs when the arteries to the kidneys are damaged. But by far the most common and tragic consequence of high blood pressure is stroke, which is a cerebrovascular accident in which either a brain artery is narrowed, a clot sticks in a narrow artery, or an artery ruptures. In any event, brain tissue is irreparably damaged, and if the person does not die, he or she may suffer significant paralysis, speech problems, or emotional disabilities.

In discussing the course of high blood pressure, Eliot makes the following point: "The time from the onset of untreated established high blood pressure to death is about twenty years. No warning signs other than a high blood pressure reading are likely to appear for about fourteen years. Then failure of one or more organs occurs. At this point, if the high blood pressure continues to go untreated, the average survival time is only about six years."[5]

There are other harmful effects of increased epinephrine and cortisol levels besides high blood pressure. These chemicals act to increase the stickiness of platelets, which are blood-clotting fragments. These sticky platelets are then more likely to adhere to the walls of arteries, creating attractive spots for blood fats to collect. At the same time, epinephrine actually creates injury in the arterial walls by scarring them, thus creating ideal places for blood fats to lodge and build up. Through these two processes, narrowing and hardening of the arteries occurs. Blood flow to the heart is compromised, and the gripping pain of angina pectoris may result. The next step may be a heart attack, in which the death of heart muscle may occur. Excessive epinephrine can also create a situation in which muscle damage occurs directly; moreover, it can cause electrical instability in the heart rhythm.

Cortisol, in contrast, seems to be related to more long-term effects. With high levels of cortisol, sodium is retained in the body tissues, more fats such as cholesterol are circulated, clotting agents are released into the blood, gastric acid secretions are increased, the production of sex hormones is decreased, and the functioning of the immune system is weakened so that the body is less able to defend itself.

The biochemistry of stress creates a significant alteration inside our body. A pattern is created whereby stress begins to feed off itself. The effects of our chronic internal imbalance produce emotional upset and physical discomfort, which, in turn, act as additional stressors; we often worry and react to our stress symptoms in a way that sets off further stress. Epinephrine and cortisol are very potent hormones, useful and helpful if produced at the right time and in the right amount—but if their levels are excessive, serious side effects may result. The situation is analogous to taking a potent pain killer or other powerful drug: in the right circumstances, the drug can be a wonderful helper, but if used excessively, unfortunate side effects can ensue. We must concede that the stress response is truly symphonic, but if it is played too frequently and too intensely, the harmony disappears, inner cacophony ensues, and ultimately the dynamic symphony of life is converted into a funeral dirge.

The Causes of Stress

Stress begins with our reaction to an event. Some efforts have been made to determine what types of external events typically initiate stress responding. Important work in this area was done by Thomas Holmes and R.H. Rahe.[6] They analyzed the relationship between the amount of life change and illness. They found that as the amount of life change increases, and the changes are more significant—such as a death in the family or a divorce—the probability of illness increases. The changes may even be of a positive nature, such as buying a house, moving, or taking a new job. Life changes demand a response; they set off emotional arousal, activate the stress response, and produce the type of internal wear and tear that leads to illness. Not everyone is equally liable to illness from life change, and certainly genetic heritage, personality characteristics, and social support systems influence the degree to which life changes will affect a person. Nevertheless, if we are experiencing a great number of life changes we can expect that we are more prone to excessive stress responding. In such situations we need to make definite efforts to manage our stress.

It is of interest to consider, however, that major life changes may create problems by the manner in which they affect our daily life. Such life changes often bring about disruptions in our normal routine, introduce frustrations, and bring forth psychological conflict, so that within the context of our daily life we are evolving more frequent and intense fight or flight responding. Richard Lazarus and his colleagues[7] have found that the number of daily hassles we experience are directly connected to our stress levels. Specifically, they discovered that if our daily hassles leave us with the sense of having too much to do, or concerns about our physical condition, the experience of losing or misplacing things or money worries or anxieties about our environment, we will encounter greater stress. In other words, if our daily life becomes disorganized and laden with worries and conflict, we have another cause of excessive stress.

Another way to consider the causes of stress is to utilize the categories of environmental stressors, physical stressors, and psychological stressors. Examples of environmental stressors are harmful chemicals (additives in our food, pollutants in the air), excessive and disturbing noises, and extremes in temperature. Such environmental stressors were used by Selye in his original experiments with animals and were found to be significant causes of stress. Certainly, we can easily appreciate the effect that loud traffic, or the constant ringing of a telephone, or an endlessly barking dog, or a day of inhaling stinging smog has on our stress levels.

Physical stressors are those produced by our bodily condition. If we are overweight, undernourished, out of shape, or have a chronic health problem, this will contribute to our stress. Such negative physical factors make direct demands on our body. Also, we must realize that environmental and physical factors interact. For example, exposure to air pollutants may lead to such physical stressors as sinusitis and a chronic sore throat, or, on the other hand, poor conditioning and habits of shallow breathing may make us more vulnerable to air pollution.

Psychological stressors interact with both environmental and physical stressors. For instance, it is common to react to noise with anger, or to react to our excessive weight with frustration and hopelessness. These emotional reactions quickly create our stress, and maintain and exacerbate our stress levels. It is indeed our psychological reaction to life changes, to daily hassles, and to environmental and physical stressors, that ultimately determines our stress levels. There are also some purely psychological causes of stress—for example, worrying about the past, about the future, or even worrying about being emotionally upset. In fact, the psychological causes of stress are so important that we must consider them in greater detail.

The Psychology of Stress

In the area of psychological stressors we can look at two distinct psychological styles that predispose us to suffer from stress. The first of these is known as the Type A personality, and the second is called the "helpless/hopeless" personality. The Type A, or coronary-prone, behavior pattern was first identified by two cardiologists, Meyer Friedman and Ray H. Rosenman,[8] who noted that many of their heart patients displayed a particular approach to life. The cardinal characteristic of this approach was an excessive struggle against time; the Type A person struggles to do more and more in less and less time. As a result, he or she walks fast, eats fast, talks fast and explosively, and feels impatient when things move slowly or when he or she has to wait in line. Type A individuals are highly competitive, especially with other Type A's; they feel vaguely guilty if they are doing nothing; and they often have a great deal of underlying hostility that explodes when they are frustrated. They focus excessively on their work and fail to notice and enjoy other facets of the environment. They become preoccupied with numbers for measuring their own self-worth.

In essence, the Type A person is engaged in a ceaseless struggle with time, and this chronic sense of struggle results in an emotional state that acts to constantly activate the fight or flight response. As a result, the Type A person typically has higher levels of muscular tension, excessive discharge of the sympathetic nervous system, and his or her blood is flooded with stress chemicals. Accordingly, Friedman and Rosenman found that Type A patients are three times as likely to experience heart disease as individuals free from Type A characteristics.

The Type A approach to life is very common in our society; it is a set of behaviors and attitudes easily learned in today's culture. The Type A lifestyle is often associated with success; people commonly feel it is the way to get ahead in life and to achieve. But, in fact, other individuals get just as much done as Type A people. The Type A approach is really geared for short-term results, and over the long term, it is destructive and limiting. The second personality style that tends to exhibit stress—the "helpless/ hopeless" style—is characterized by a particularly negative mental set. The core belief here is that no matter what one does, it is not going to have much effect. In other words, one feels powerless, caught, and stuck, with no way out. One believes that he or she has no real control over the important aspects of his or her personal life, health, and environment.

Physically, the helpless/hopeless response can be quite lethal, for we are giving the body two contradictory messages. On one hand, we sense that something is wrong, and hence the body activates to deal with long-term stressors—but at the same time we conclude that nothing can be done about the situation, so we shut down and give up. This is analogous to simultaneously pushing a car's accelerator and brake. The damage can be very extensive.

Often, people fall into the helpless/hopeless mode when there is an important loss in life (for example, the death of a spouse or the loss of a job) or some other event that makes them feel that things are beyond their control. But there are also many learned factors regarding our sense of self-worth, our estimate of options and solutions, and our evaluation of life tragedies that can predispose us to this state of hopelessness. The psychology of hopelessness and its physiological consequences are described in detail in Chapter 11 of this book, entitled "Stress, Helplessness, and Hope." Suffice it to say at this point that the hopeless/helpless personality is an important psychological risk factor for stress.

Habits and Stress

We must also consider the role of life habits in increasing stress. The various components of the stress response are sensitive to one another to the extent that if we, through our life habits, are continually activating one component, we will tend to get an elevation across the entire stress response. For example, if we eat junk food that is loaded with sugar, we will predictably experience a rise in blood sugar level that gives us a feeling of increased energy. This same increase is, however, also a part of the stress response. The increase in blood sugar tends to interact with other components of the stress response and set them off. So we may notice an increase in heart rate, a slight lift in blood pressure, a change in breathing, and a subtle change in the entire tone of the autonomic nervous system and the body's biochemistry. Thus, poor life habits can result in increased stress.

In the case of sugar intake, there is more involved than just an immediate effect. The sugar high is often followed by a sugar low, when the amount of insulin released by the pancreas exceeds what is required and depletes the blood sugar level. The result is a so-called hypoglycemia attack, in which symptoms of dizziness, irritability, depression, tremor, nausea, and anxiety may occur. Such an attack may act directly as a stressor or may impair our behavioral efficiency to the point where we create additional stressors for ourselves. The overall result is that our dietary habits have added significantly to our stress level and reduced our ability to cope. Excessive caffeine intake and alcohol consumption are other examples of habits that can compound stress.

Breathing habits tend to influence directly the autonomic nervous system and thereby have a significant impact upon our stress response pattern. If we habitually breathe too rapidly, shallowly, and thoracically, we are unintentionally creating a pattern that would normally be set off only by the flight or fight response. The body doesn't seem to be able to make the discrimination that such a breathing pattern is merely a habit and not a real emergency. Consequently, the entire autonomic chain of stress reactors is activated. Our heart rate, blood pressure, and peripheral vascular constriction are increased. Here again, we have an instance of a habit that acts to over-drive the stress response.

From the perspective of yoga, the proper regulation of breathing is seen as a direct avenue for tuning and balancing the nervous system. Several chapters in this anthology discuss breathing habits and provide guidelines for positive change.

Obviously, our postural habits, sleep habits, exercise

habits, and emotional habits can all play the same role of contributing to, interacting with, and chronically activating our stress levels. Stress is a complex pattern, diverse in its course and rich in interaction among its various physiological channels. It is a pattern that can develop its own momentum: stress weakens our ability to cope with stressors; stress produces more stressors; as a response to stress, we may develop life habits that actually increase our stress.

The Goals of Stress Management

Before beginning to try to reduce stress, it is helpful to have a clearly defined and positive view of the goals of stress management. Often, people think that the opposite of stress is relaxation. Therefore, they think that the answer to the stress problem is becoming quiet, passive, and relaxed. But then they worry that they would never get anything done that way or never achieve. So they end up believing that they need stress to keep motivated and achieving. In fact, stress management is a great deal more dynamic. Managing stress should lead not only to a reduction in stress-related symptoms but should lead as well to optimal health. By managing stress we can become more dynamic and active in life. The opposite of stress is not a passive state, but a state in which physiological, mental, and emotional resources are tuned and balanced to a level of optimum effectiveness. We can then become active in dealing with demands as they occur, yet simultaneously have the ability and skills that allow us to protect, rest, and restore our internal resources. This dynamic state is the goal in stress management.

Let us begin our practical search for this goal by considering the nature of optimal performance. It is generally accepted that there is a predictable relationship between arousal, or physiological activation, and performance. As arousal increases we perform better, up to a point where too much arousal interferes with performance.

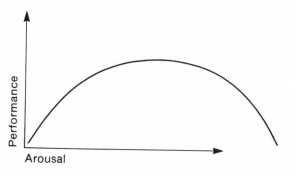

Figure 4
The Relationship Between Arousal and Performance

This relationship is portrayed in the diagram above.

Accordingly, if we are under-activated or over-activated, our performance suffers. For example, if we're half asleep we can't give a good speech; we need more energy for such an occasion. Conversely, if our heart is racing madly, our knees knocking together, our mouth dry and voice shaky, we are too nervous to give a good speech. Clearly the best solution is to match activation to the task at hand. But this appropriate matching gets harder and harder for individuals with excessive stress. They end up being chronically over-activated, their performance suffers, and the only solution they may know is to try to calm themselves down with tranquilizers or alcohol. Periodically, they may crash at levels of under-arousal, and then require stimuli to get them energized for action.

The process of matching arousal to the task at hand is a dynamic function. In 1982, Duncan Currey and the author conducted a research experiment that has some bearing on the ideal we strive for in stress management.[9] We investigated the way three different groups of people reacted to and recovered from exposure to a stressor. The three groups that we studied were: (a) chronic pain patients, (b) "normals," who were hospital staff members free from any illness and not taking medication, and (c) "relaxers," who were people who had practiced some form of relaxation at least five times a week for a minimum of a year. We measured forehead muscle tension and fingertip temperature. The former is a good measure of the amount of muscular bracing and tension; the latter indicates the degree of sympathetic ANS activity. Each subject was given five minutes to relax, and was then challenged with the mental task of subtracting by sevens from 1,000 out loud as quickly as possible. Most people find this a stressful task. Finally, in the recovery stage, we gave them another five minutes to relax.

Our findings with regard to muscle tension were initially very much as we expected: the pain patients had more tension, more activation when exposed to stress, and less ability to recover. The normal subjects showed basically the same pattern but at less extreme level. The relaxers showed the least tension and had the quickest recovery, but they also showed something quite surprising during the stressor phase. In the first 90 seconds of the math task, they displayed a faster and more dramatic *increase* in muscular activity than the other two groups, after which their tension levels quickly dropped and leveled off. This pattern can be seen in the diagram below.

Figure 5
Muscular Activation Patterns

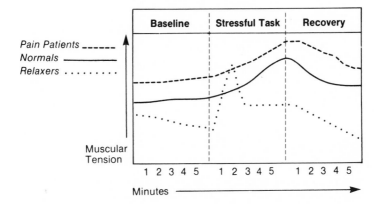

It appears that the relaxers when confronted with an environmental demand, showed a quick and dramatic activation. However, they also automatically adjusted their level of activation once they caught on to the task. The relaxers behaved in a surprising manner; we expected them simply to be more relaxed all the way through. They indeed showed lower levels of tension, but they also showed a more dynamic, appropriate, and flexible response. Our subjective analysis of what the relaxers experienced suggested that they shifted to what might be called a right-brain strategy. That is they closed their eyes and visualized a pattern of numbers and scanned down the pattern rather than trying to subtract by seven each time. This is an effective problem-solving approach that would be difficult to use if one was too tense. They needed to relax a little to utilize this strategy.

The relaxers had apparently developed a very useful and healthy mechanism. They could activate their resources quickly to meet a challenge, but then readjust as soon as they determined the amount of activation required for the task at hand. When the task was completed, they were quickly able to return to a relaxed level. The relaxers in our study were simply more efficient, more flexible, and more dynamic. They apparently had developed a mechanism both for keeping themselves in the optimum range of the performance curve and for not wasting energy. This gives us some insight into the nature of effective stress management.

There may be biochemical correlates of this flexibility. Research conducted by Dr. Robert Sapolsky on baboons (primates with a stress mechanism similar to humans) found that baboons ranking high in a stable social hierarchy had a different biochemical stress response than those lower in the hierarchy.[10] Sapolsky looked in particular at cortisol, a hormone secreted by the adrenal gland under the direction of the brain and pituitary gland. As mentioned earlier, cortisol is a key component of the stress response chemistry that converts sugar into blood glucose, influences the functioning of the brain, and inhibits reproduction, growth, and immune functioning. High-ranking baboons had lower resting levels of cortisol, yet they responded to environmental challenges with a faster and longer increase in cortisol levels. Moreover, they were able to switch off the cortisol more rapidly. As Sapolsky notes: "Thus, high-ranking males responded to stress with the fastest rises in cortisol but had the lowest levels of this potent hormone circulating at all other times, when its effect is harmful rather than useful."[11]

If we begin to regard this pattern of general physiological stability coupled with response flexibility as a goal of stress management, then we must examine the mechanism or process that encourages such a response profile. In this inquiry the model of a negative feedback system, as described in systems theory, can be quite useful. A negative feedback system is characterized by stability and balance. The classic example of a negative feedback system is the heating and cooling system in a building. Typically such a system may work to maintain temperatures at an optimal range between 68 and 72 degrees. If the temperature rises above 72 degrees the thermostat will register the increasing temperature and switch on the air conditioning so that the temperature is brought back into the desired range. Conversely, when the temperature drops below 68 degrees, the thermostat registers the decreasing temperature and switches on the heating system.

Thus, by receiving negative feedback that the temperature is out of the ideal range, the system activates the appropriate heating or cooling unit to bring the temperature back into the desired range. Two components are needed to make this system work. The first is sensitivity, for the thermometer must be sensitive to changes in temperature. The second is control, because the system must be able to control or move the temperature up or down.

If we apply this negative feedback model to humans and the problem of stress, a number of things become clear. First of all, stress-related illness occurs when our negative feedback system gets out of balance. That is, the body, in fact, gets overheated, or undercooled, or fluctuates wildly between the two. If we desire to reduce stress we must rediscover and then refine the two critical processes of sensitivity and control. We must learn to become sensitive, to be aware when our body is being over-driven: to notice the strain in our breath, the excessive muscular tension, and the driving of our heart, and to feel the effect of the hormones our body produces under excessive stress. When we note these various manifestations of overheating, we must be able to implement effective control and regulation strategies that work with the mind, emotions, body, and breath to cool the system down and reachieve balance. Conversely, we must also be sensitive to overcooling in our system—able to notice the mental hopelessness, stifled breathing, physical lethargy, and any faltering of the immune system—and be able to energize and restore our system to a healthy level.

Much of stress management, then, is a progression of learning, or perhaps relearning, and then constantly refining our skills of inner sensitivity and control. We need to become "insiders", that is, we need to work on cultivating a highly developed inner awareness and control. For an adept insider, the possibility of being one of the sufferers of a "silent epidemic" or of falling prey to an unknown malady is as ludicrous as failing to notice an open window in winter or an oven left on in summer. But the reality is that we have learned to ignore vital information coming from within. If we have a headache, stomachache, backache, anxiety attack, or a period of fatigue, we want to get rid of the symptom, instead of viewing it as vital, useful feedback. We go for the short-term fix and reach for aspirin or other pain killer rather than trying to understand what has created the imbalance. In a similar manner we look to such stimulants as coffee, sweets, tobacco, and alcohol to keep us going when we feel tired or worn out. We ignore, suppress, or misinterpret the signals from within that are trying to make us aware that some rebalancing, some inner adjustments, are needed. As a consequence, the problem of stress is compounded; we go from bad to worse.

We need to develop a personal philosophy that encourages the flourishing of inner awareness and self-regulation. We need to appreciate the various signs and symptoms of being overheated or undercooled as vital and useful information. We should assign a high priority to creating those conditions whereby we can learn and refine our inner skills. For instance, we can learn to use periods of exercise, relaxation, cleansing, and silence as the staging area for developing these vital skills of self-regulation.

The stress response can be an appropriate and useful short-term response to a situation or condition. But if the stress response is overused and abused, it clearly leads to illness and lowered efficiency. For the long haul, self-regulation is the most appropriate response. It allows us to protect our health and to enhance our efficiency. If we are in balance, we can respond appropriately to significant stressors when they arise.

Another positive goal of stress management has to do with enhancing performance in a rather direct manner. For, as we have already noted, the cumulative effects of stress tend to decrease mental efficiency—memory, concentration, perceptual acuity, decision making, and creative thinking. As these skills are inhibited and decreased, the instances in which they fail are situations that create stress. For example, the time when we just can't concentrate or can't remember important information may create frustration and anger or may lead us to make a significant mistake. Either of these outcomes leads to more stress, which further impairs our mental skills and contributes to a general pattern of increasing frustration and ineffectiveness.

By contrast, many of the techniques used in stress management—such as relaxation, exercise, breath regulation, diet, and meditation—work directly and indirectly to improve our mental skills. For example, after practicing relaxation we typically experience greater mental clarity. We see, hear, feel, taste, and touch more accurately and more sensitively. Similarly, after exercise and a release of tension, it is common to experience an improved ability to reason, to think intuitively, and to make decisions. Moreover, proper diet can provide the raw materials needed by the nervous system to function properly. We experience the result as mental clarity. Meditation, as described later in this book, is an extremely useful technique that works on many levels of mental functioning. Through the practice of meditation unconscious conflicts are released, the mind becomes clearer, and intuition is strengthened. As a result we find our mind to be a more useful tool. The regular practice of breathing exercises also allows the mind to function more smoothly and effectively.

These various stress management techniques act in a palliative or treatment sense. They reduce the adverse effects of stress and bring us back to our natural baseline of mental efficiency. As we are able to utilize our intellectual potential, it is also likely that we prevent additional stress. We are better able to avoid unwise and stress-causing decisions and excessive negative emotional reactions. Finally, as we continue to practice these techniques, we move into another phase, one of direct enhancement of mental skills. Through the practice of stress management skills we begin to directly improve our mental skills. Memory, concentration, perceptual acuity, intuition, and reasoning improve, and are more available for us when we need them. This direct enhancement of mental skills is an additional positive outcome of stress management.

So far in our discussion we have established flexibility, self-regulation, and enhanced mental performance as goals for a stress management program. There is still one ingredient missing. In describing human functioning it is as if we have been talking about a machine, as though the human body were a splendid automobile that we want to maintain in mint condition. But this is an entirely too mechanical approach. There is more to health than a fit machine. If we inquire within we might realize that being healthy allows us to do the things we want to do in life. Health becomes a means or a vehicle that allows us to work toward our goals in life. Health allows us to unfold our potentials and to progress toward an ever-deepening understanding of life.

It is in this context that stress management becomes something living and exciting. We introduce the factor of intention into our life. We have the goal of self unfoldment, and health is one of the means to reach that goal. Stress is an impediment. Interestingly enough, if we desire to be healthy our physiology responds. It is similar to what occurred as infants when we decided that we wanted to walk. Our muscles, nervous system, and perceptual systems all cooperated in learning a very complex and useful pattern, that of ambulation. Freedom from stress can also be a goal. Ultimately our physical systems respond to the clarity of our intent and they can learn the complex skills of self-regulation.

The intensity of our desire for health is related to how clear we are about our direction in life. Simply stated, this means that when we have a clear sense of purpose in life we recognize that we need health to achieve this purpose. Therefore, the more clarity we have about our purpose in life and our specific goals, the more energy will come into our efforts at stress management. With such clarity it becomes important to make being healthy a priority, and consequently our conscious and unconscious mind find the resources needed to reduce stress and enhance health. Increasing clarity about our goals in life is then another component of effective stress management.

Along these lines there is one final consideration that must be brought forward. We cannot equate health and minimal stress only with a healthy body. For there can be situations in which we have a chronic illness, a genetically based disability, the consequences of an injury or the results of earlier stress. Does the existence of such problems mean that we are doomed to be a failure in terms of stress management? Probably not. For we must realize that there is a level of mental and spiritual wellness that is independent of our physical health. Freedom from stress is a state of mind and an inner experience. Even in the face of a chronic disability we can have an innate sense of satisfaction, contentment, and appreciation of life. This is an inner state of basic healthiness, and this basic healthiness is another goal of stress management.

In summary, we may keep in mind that there are a number of components involved in stress management. These include learning to be flexible and appropriate in our response to stressors and maintaining physiological balance. It has to do with obtaining higher levels of creativity and personal effectiveness. It includes clarity about our goals in life. Ultimately it means achieving a basic internal state of health, a mental and spiritual state of well-being that allows us to express our finest potentials.

With these goals in mind, we are ready to begin the journey of practical stress management and learn the specific skills of inner awareness and self-regulation that are described in the following chapters. Stress is a pattern that perpetuates itself and develops its own momentum. Hence, we must first learn to slow this momentum, to stop making things worse, to stop feeding the stress cycle. Often, revising harmful habits, reducing muscular tension, and changing thought patterns and emotions can help in slowing the stress cycle. At the same time, we have the opportunity to establish another pattern, one of increasing health, that may gain momentum over time. As we continually refine our inner awareness and develop the ability to control our body, we have an increasing experience of a natural state of health. We become more aware of subtle habits that may be nudging us off balance and of deeper emotional patterns that are unproductive. We can learn to change these harmful habits and patterns, and as we reduce them, we may discover that our application of stress reduction techniques becomes more refined and more effective. Now, let us explore these skills and techniques.

CHAPTER 2
Stress, Exercise and Relaxation

John Clarke, M.D.

Physical exercise has a unique and beneficial role to play in helping us to relax and in counteracting the effects of sustained day-to-day stress. Aerobic exercise, such as jogging, and the postures of hatha yoga are complementary in their effects on releasing tension from the body, especially on one of the major physical reservoirs of stress—the musculo-skeletal system. To understand how these systems of exercise can be effective in the management of stress, it is helpful to review what stress is and how its consequences arise, particularly in the development of excessive muscular tension.

As described in the previous chapter by Dr. Harvey, stress has been characterized as a set of internal responses to the environment that leads to a state of imbalance, requiring us to expend energy, consciously or unconsciously, to restore our balance. Designated as *homeostasis* by Walter Bradford Cannon, an early researcher, this tendency to return to an equilibrium point can be illustrated by examining the result of our exposure to cold. When we are exposed to cold, our body temperature falls and we

Reprinted from Dawn *magazine, Vol. 2, Number 2, 1982*

activate innate physical mechanisms that both conserve heat by reduction in blood flow to the skin and increase the production of body heat—for instance, by shivering. These reflexes may restore the temperature imbalance and return our low body heat to normal, but they do so at the expense of realignment of blood flow and by additional muscular activity. As the body temperature approaches normal, the shivering may stop, but the blood flow is still shunted away from the skin and extremities, which can lead to cold, painful, or even frostbitten fingers or toes. The degree of physical stress experienced in this situation may be difficult to measure. The body temperature may be normal, there may be no shivering, and the degree of blood redistribution may be noticeable only in comparison with a previous baseline state; but a temperature stress is nonetheless being experienced, and an attempt to restore equilibrium, or to adapt, is occurring.

So, on a physical level, an environmental change—if it influences the body—can lead to an imbalance, a deviation from the body's equilibrium, which automatically activates innate mechanisms in an attempt to restore the equilibrium. Energy is required for this, and less energy is consequently available for other activities or for responses to other stresses. The degree of energy required to adapt depends, first, on how much the stress affects us; second, on how long its effects on us last; and, third, on how frequently it occurs. In the case of cold exposure, for instance, we can insulate ourselves with clothing so that even extremely cold temperatures have minimal influence on us.

Most of the common physical stresses in our lives are no longer the stresses associated with survival, but are more subtle, less obvious physical stresses, such as improper lighting, high ambient noise, poor quality of air and food, overcrowding, subsonic vibrations associated with motor vehicles, and other concomitants of our technologically advanced culture.

The most common stressors in our present environment, however, are not physical but mental. These stressors, then, are an important focus for stress management. The sequence of events occurring with mental stress is similar to that occurring with physical stress. At the most general level, any event, internal or external, that creates a change in our internal environment—physical, emotional, or mental—can be viewed as a stressor. In a somewhat oversimplified description, the appearance of a thought or mental image in our mind automatically creates a readiness in our body to undertake activities that have become associated with that image. For instance, if we think of a lemon, our mouth automatically begins to produce saliva and our intestines become more active. Similarly, if we know we are about to exert ourselves physically, our breath and heart rate become more active, even if we are still sitting quietly.

These responses occur automatically through both our nervous system and our glandular system. The part of the nervous system associated with this response is called the involuntary nervous system, as distinct from the voluntary nervous system, which is responsible for activating our skeletal muscles to carry out our desired movements. This latter system is called "voluntary" because we have learned consciously how to use it, although the actual way we use our muscles is non-conscious. It may well be that the functions of the involuntary nervous system could become more voluntary if we understood better how to work with them.

This involuntary nervous system is known as the autonomic nervous system and has two branches, the sympathetic nervous system (SNS) and the parasympathetic nervous system (PNS). The crucial role and function of the sympathetic and parasympathetic nervous systems have been explained in the previous chapter by Dr. Harvey. Yet when we consider the issue of tension there are several aspects of the SNS that bear careful consideration and particular emphasis. The SNS tends to become activated when we have to act in the external world, that is, when we perceive events in a way that requires an external action or response on our part—such as speech or physical action— particularly if the external events are perceived as threatening our own personal psychological or physical security or well-being. The full response of the SNS in its role of mobilizing our energy to protect ourselves from a life-threatening danger has best been characterized by Cannon. He termed this activation the "fight or flight response," suggesting that animals, when attacked, would either need to stand and fight or to run away. With regard to the physical body, both responses impose similar muscular, cardiorespiratory, and energy requirements.

The responses that we commonly term stressful are associated with SNS activity. There are two characteristics of the SNS that make us particularly susceptible to its excessive activity. The first is that it is designed, when activated, to respond quickly and fully. If we are in a sudden danger that requires a rapid response, we need the capability to mobilize our energy and quickly put ourselves into activity. The second property, concomitant with the first, is that the SNS is patterned in a way such as to react throughout the whole body, putting all of our body activities on alert. Both of these characteristics are distinct from the operation of the parasympathetic nervous system, which has a slower, more graded onset of action and more localized effects.

We have all experienced—in response to a startling noise or a clear threat—the sensations of instant alertness, pounding heart, and muscle tension, all from a sudden, strong, generalized reaction of the SNS. This characteristic of the SNS is important—and, for animals, oftentimes life-saving—but is an inheritance from our ancestors. Most of our present-day stressors are not physical or immediate.

Seldom do they require a massive physical response. However, just as we may overreact to a sudden noise that proves to be short-lived and harmless, so also may we overreact to any stressor in our life, or our reaction may long outlast the precipitating events.

Anatomy of Tension

Overreactivity and *prolonged or incomplete recovery,* then, are the problems of importance in managing stress. These problems can be seen more clearly by considering what occurs after we mentally perceive and decide that some event is threatening. In such an instance there is an automatic response through the ANS to put our body "on guard," and part of this response involves nerve impulses being transmitted to appropriate muscles, to contract them to create a movement or action. If for some reason we decide to inhibit or stop this action (as is often the case), another impulse is then sent to an opposing muscle group to prevent motion. So that now, to prevent a certain action from taking place, two opposing sets of muscles have unnecessary tension in them. The greater our impulse to move, the more tension must go into the opposing muscle group to keep us motionless. In this tense motionless state, the nerve and muscle cells are active and using energy needlessly, while the blood flow, carrying its supply of replacement energy, is decreased because of the effect of muscle contraction compressing the blood vessels. The same motionlessness that occurs in the tense state could occur were there no activity in either muscle group (that is, complete relaxation), but the overall physical effects would be entirely different.

Tension begins to accumulate in this fashion in the body. Then, as we face the challenges of daily living, the SNS activity tends to reinforce this pattern of tension. Tension in our body can foster a state of mental tension, which in turn creates more physical tension, and a vicious cycle can ensue. The breathing pattern can also reflect and exacerbate this state of over-arousal and tension. This state of tension can increase, not only on a daily basis, but over weeks, months, and even years. Muscle tension then represents the residual in the muscles of mental impulses toward action that have become blocked or inhibited. How can the cycle be broken, and relaxation established?

We need to find a way to develop ourselves so that our reaction to stress involves a response appropriate to the stimulus, in degree as well as in duration. Because residual tension in us sensitizes us to new stress, and can lead to excessive and prolonged responses ("our nerves are on edge"), the most efficient place for most of us to begin in the control of stress is with release of tension currently present in individual muscle groups. To release this chronic muscular tension and its associated contraction, three avenues of approach are available: working directly with the muscles themselves, working with the breath, and working with the mind and its activity. These categories are not mutually exclusive (for instance, helping the mind relax will affect the tension in the muscles, and vice versa) but represent areas of primary emphasis and attention. To work directly with the muscles in reducing chronic tension, both exercise and certain relaxation techniques can be used. Two useful, complementary approaches to physical exercise are aerobics and hatha yoga.

Since tension, particularly muscular tension, represents an unreleased impulse to act, we can give expression to that blocked energy by muscular activity. Jogging or brisk walking may be particularly effective ways to do this because they are very similar to the basic type of activity for which the SNS seems programmed—that is, to run, either in attack or in flight. Another way to release tension physically is to *stretch* the muscles, and that is the principle underlying hatha yoga. Because opposing muscle groups often carry equivalent tension, it is important, as a general principle, to stretch muscles first in one direction and then in the opposite. So exercise can be effective in reducing tension in two ways: first by *expressing* the impulse underlying the tension through muscular activity, such as aerobic exercise; and second, by *releasing* the tension and contraction through stretching techniques, such as hatha yoga. Let us now consider each of these approaches in greater detail.

Aerobic exercise takes its name from activity that occurs in the presence of air (oxygen, to be specific). In contrast, *anaerobic* exercise occurs in the relative absence of oxygen. Anaerobic activity usually occurs because the demands we are placing on a group of muscles exceed our ability to supply them with oxygen from the bloodstream. There is no sharp cutoff between these two categories. The functional difference is that in anaerobic activity, lactic acid builds up in the bloodstream; in fact, the amount of lactic acid buildup can be used as a measure of the degree to which an activity is anaerobic.

Perhaps the most useful guide to determining the anaerobic component of exertion is the ease of breathing. If our breathing pattern is even and comfortable, allowing us to carry on a conversation if we wish, then it is well within our aerobic capacity. A marked acceleration or deepening of respiration, with a sense of not being able to get quite enough air, suggests that we have exerted ourselves beyond our aerobic capacity.

The physical responses to aerobic exercise are of interest because of their close relationship to the stress response. As we increase our exertion to maximum, the amount of oxygen taken into the body can be measured and is found to increase in direct proportion to the level of our exertion, as might be expected. As we reach our capacity, however, the level of oxygen intake reaches a maximum and plateaus; no longer able to increase with increased intensity of exertion, and our efforts become anaerobic. The level at which this occurs is designated the "VO_2 max," signifying technically the maximum oxygen uptake per minute—that is, our aerobic capacity. It is a consistent value for each of us, yet one that can vary significantly from person to person and probably has a strong genetic component. Olympic athletes trained in long distance running, cross-country skiing, or crew races have the highest values of VO_2 max (in the range of 60-80 cc of O_2/kg min). Aging appears inexorably to reduce our capacity about 1 cc of O_2 per year. Training can increase our capacity about twenty percent, and may decrease the rate at which it falls with age.

As we exercise more strenuously, there is a close parallel between the degree of activation of the SNS and the level of oxygen uptake (VO_2). If we are jogging at fifty percent of our maximal aerobic capacity (50% of VO_2 max), then our SNS is also activated at about fifty percent of its maximal capacity. In aerobic exercise, the heart rate is an excellent guide to sympathetic activity, and it, too, increases gradually to a maximum plateau, just as does VO_2. So a convenient way to measure the degree of SNS activation (as well as to gauge where we are in terms of our maximum aerobic capacity), is simply to measure our pulse rate, at any level of exertion, and compare it to its maximum value.

Our maximum heart rate falls with age, and can be estimated by subtracting our age from 205 or 210. Thus, a fifty-year-old man would have an estimated maximum heart rate of between 155 and 160 beats per minute. If he noticed a heart rate of 120 while walking, he would know that he was exerting himself at approximately seventy-five percent of his maximal capacity. This is useful to know because many of the physical benefits of walking or jogging appear to occur only if the intensity of exercise is high enough. This "training effect" appears to occur at exercise levels intense enough to stimulate the heart rate sixty to eighty percent of its maximum. For most of us, that is a heart rate in the range of 110 to 140 beats per minute, depending upon our age. More frequent exercise sessions at this intensity, especially for people just beginning a program, lead to an increased risk of injury due to inadequate rest and recovery time. The exercise program itself then becomes a source of significant, if unperceived, stress.

Obviously, though, individual strengths and capacities vary greatly, and the best guideline as to how much exercise to do is whether one feels progressively better overall and is increasingly free from discomfort, or whether significant aches and pains or progressive fatigue occurs, making it more and more difficult to awaken or move about, particularly on arising in the morning. Proper aerobic training has been shown to have many significant benefits, both psychological and physical. Decreased tension and anxiety (to the degree that the use of tranquilizers becomes unnecessary) has been demonstrated, as well as increased spontaneity, creativity, and self-confidence. Some have even reported a "jogger's high"—a sense of euphoria that can develop after a prolonged run. Exercise at this level of intensity, lasting twenty to thirty minutes, three to five times a week, also appears to be the most efficient way to condition the cardiovascular system, and achieve what is called a "training effect."

The physical benefits of this exercise include a lower resting heart rate (the hallmark of the training effect), a lowered blood pressure, a reduction in weight, and changes in the chemical composition of the blood, such as decreases in blood sugar and in total cholesterol and triglyceride levels, and an increased level of HDL-cholesterol—a blood component that is thought to protect against heart disease. The interesting feature of these changes is that they correspond for the most part with a decreased level of SNS activity. How is it that exercise, which stimulates the SNS, can be associated with an overall reduction of SNS activity?

Recommending exercise as a treatment of stress might at first seem like adding fuel to the fire. Certainly, some persons can overdo exercise and create additional stress, but for most of us, it is of positive benefit. Activation of sympathetic activity through this type of exertion appears to release somewhat the chronic activation developed by stress.

Both brisk walking and long slow jogging are excellent techniques of aerobic exercise that help with stress reduction. The rate of exercise should be enough to stimulate an increase in rate and depth of breath without creating a sense of breathlessness. For maximum safety, an exercise stress test, under medical supervision, should be taken by anyone thirty years or older who is initiating an aerobic exercise program.

While jogging or walking, breathe through the nose. This will not only stimulate the entire respiratory mechanism but will act as a governor to prevent overexertion. When you need to breathe through the mouth, you may be pushing yourself too much. Try to practice a sustained awareness of your breathing and muscular effort as you jog or walk. Watch for physical tension and breathing irregularities and observe your mental patterns. A few minutes of loosening up exercises before and after the jogging are also helpful.

But many of the benefits of exercise, particularly the psychological benefits and an increased sense of well-being, can be achieved at levels of exertion that are much less intense than seventy or eighty percent of our maximal capacity. Brisk walking, for instance, has long been recommended by physicians, and has an increasing number of enthusiastic advocates. It is much less jarring on the bones and joints than jogging, and creates less undesired muscle tightness. It has been shown to be effective, as well, in weight loss programs, and is less likely to create sudden heart problems. Just walking around a lot during the day, however, does not seem to yield the greatest benefits. The walking should be a separate activity, carried out at a brisk, rhythmic pace, sustained continuously for twenty to thirty minutes, preferably outdoors, with attention given to a regular, relaxed pattern of diaphragmatic breathing through the nose. Walking under other conditions—such as with the family dog, with its meandering starts and stops and its need for frequent attention—will unfortunately not optimize the benefits of this form of exertion.

An interesting form of exercise that combines many of the positive aspects of both walking and jogging is what has been called Long Slow Distance ("LSD") jogging. This type of jogging features a slower pace, one at which a conversation can be maintained. It has helped people avoid going beyond their capacity. Injuries have decreased, and the pleasant aspects of the process of exercise, such as conversation with a friend, or enjoying the scenery, are emphasized more than the issues of training, competition, or goal-attainment. Running is then more enjoyable and people's motivation to continue is more easily sustained. The mind becomes freed from constant attention to training protocols and goals. The slow jog is very far removed from high-intensity training. The pace may be slower than a walk, and could approach or include running in place. Using this technique still allows people to achieve a training effect, however, even to the point of running in marathons. The psychological milieu of slow jogging can entirely remove many of the self-competitive aspects of running, such as an emphasis on distance covered or duration of time at a higher level of effort. It is often quite instructive to try to run as *slowly* as possible, and notice at what point a sense of impatience or frustration emerges—the feeling of not getting anywhere. All of the elements that can lead to the enjoyment of running are present, except the idea of getting somewhere.

Pushing ourselves at a level close to our limits is a

habit that can often characterize the way we approach many, if not most, of our activities of life. We often are unwilling to allow the enjoyment of the process of doing something to take precedence over the achievement of a goal. Slow jogging can help us begin to decrease the attitude of constant self-pushing, of constantly forcing ourselves to improve or excel. As this begins to happen, an interesting experience may emerge. As we slow down and stop trying to keep a certain pace or reach a certain distance, much more of our awareness is free to be directed to the natural surroundings, or to more subtle aspects of the activity of jogging, and a process of inner exploration can begin. One can work, for instance, with varying patterns of breathing and notice the effects of varying the pattern—such as using a more full, active exhalation or prolonging the exhalation to twice the duration of inhalation, or prolonging the duration of the entire breath. At faster paces, this is often uncomfortable.

In addition, areas of excessive muscular tension, often overlooked, can become more apparent. Excessive tension often accumulates in the muscles of the arms, the neck, the abdomen, and even the legs themselves, and can lead to inefficient performance as well as injury. Slowing one's pace to a crawl can help create a setting in which it is easier to identify these areas, to become more sensitive to them, and to learn to relax them consciously.

Hatha yoga stands in somewhat an analogous position to calisthenics as slow jogging does to conventional aerobics: in both hatha and slow jogging there are quiet, slower movements with an emphasis on an increased awareness of the inner sensations associated with the activity being performed. There are empirical studies in the literature of physical therapy, for instance, that give support to the efficacy of stretching techniques using the principles of hatha. Performing regular calisthenics can be invigorating and does lead to "warming up" and "loosening up," but can also have a potentially harsh, jarring quality, which leaves little room or time for the mind to become increasingly subtle or sensitive in its awareness of inner activity. The slow, sustained stretch in hatha allows for a much greater awareness of the inner realm of body sensations, as well as of breathing patterns.

Doing from fifteen to forty-five minutes of stretching exercise per day is quite beneficial. The postures or asanas of hatha yoga are ideal in this regard. These asanas are designed to stretch complementary sets of muscles in a gradual and complete manner. The basic asanas and some gentle introductory stretches are described in *Hatha Yoga Manual I* and *Joints and Glands Exercises,* books published by the Himalayan Institute.

It may also be helpful to take a hatha yoga class to ensure that the postures are learned correctly. Once you have a good knowledge of yoga asanas, you can choose a routine each day that meets your needs. As with the aerobic exercises, awareness and attention to the breathing and muscular effort are crucial. Pay attention to all levels of your being when you perform the postures. Regulate your breathing, concentrate your mind, and gently stretch out any tension buildup. At the conclusion of your hatha practice, do a brief relaxation. Also, some of the joint and gland exercises, such as neck rolls and shoulder lifts, can be performed occasionally during the day to prevent tension from accumulating.

Rehabilitation experts who work with stroke or cerebral palsy patients with very tense, spastic muscles have found that the most effective or efficient way to relax these muscles is through a slow, sustained stretch, just strong enough that a sensation of stretch occurs, but mild enough that no pain or discomfort occurs. It must be a mild stretch, because if discomfort occurs, unconscious protective reflexes are triggered in the body to protect the muscles from further stretching, which causes them to contract.

Thus, if stretched excessively, the muscles resist, by reflex, the very progress one is trying to make.

This reflexive tensing of muscles in the presence of pain is analogous to the response that occurs when we react to a perceived stress, and is accompanied and markedly accentuated by breath irregularities, particularly breath holding or apnea. The emphasis that is placed in hatha yoga on the maintenance of a slow, deep, even respiration during postures facilitates the process of muscular relaxation and stretching. Because of the relationship between breath and ANS functioning, the relaxation effect takes place not only in the muscles but throughout the body. In light of this, it has been speculated that many of the beneficial effects of sustained, continuous aerobic exercise come not only from the improved circulation of blood through the body but from the effects of the sustained, regular, even flow of breathing stimulated by the need for increased oxygen and carbon dioxide exchange.

Viewing exercise in the context of stress management highlights its value in reducing tension and anxiety and in facilitating relaxation. This may appear to be somewhat paradoxical because, although many of us would readily admit that exercise helps us relax, we tend to think of relaxation techniques themselves as being quiet and motionless rather than active. The dimension of relaxation during exercise, particularly aerobic exercise, has been given relatively little attention, except indirectly in the suggestion to perform stretching exercises in the warming up and cooling down times around the exercise period. Unnecessarily tense muscles expend energy needlessly, and do not receive as much blood flow as possible.

The system of hatha yoga reflects this awareness in its emphasis on periods of time devoted specifically to relaxation at the end of a practice session and between individual postures, as well as in its emphasis on breath-related relaxation during the maintenance of each posture. When we use our muscles to exert ourselves, particularly as the degree of effort increases, there is a natural tendency to "tense up" and contract muscles not involved in the exertion itself. A common example of this is the tension in the fingers created when writing with pen or pencil. For many, the muscle tension is far more than is necessary to stabilize the pen for writing, and can even lead to finger, joint, and arm pain. As people become aware of this, and consciously relax the excessive tension, a shift in the appearance of the writing often occurs, toward a more open, light, and fluid style.

Conscious synchronization of the breath with body movement while relaxing areas of tension can help reduce this tendency toward excessive muscular tension. Breath irregularities, on the other hand, particularly breath holding, can make the tendency worse. To become sensitized to the excessive buildup during exercise of muscular tension—a manifestation of stress in itself—it is instructive to become familiar with (as well as to practice) some techniques of relaxation.

Focused Relaxation

Full relaxation and release of tension take place best when the significant factors associated with tension are directly and consciously taken into account. These include the muscular system, the circulatory system (as an expression of ANS activity), the breathing pattern, the activity of the mind, and our habitual psychological attitudes. It is necessary for the tension in the muscles to be released, the extremities to become warm, the breath to be quiet, even, and deep, and the mind's activity to be gently removed from stressful thoughts to relaxing ones, or, preferably, to guiding and observing the process of relaxation in the body. Achieving the correct posture, systematically reviewing the muscles or other parts of the body with the intent that they become relaxed, or attending to the sensation of warmth and heaviness in the limbs, can facilitate release of tension, and are commonly used relaxation techniques.

Consciously directed relaxation using the breath or other points of focus, or the relaxation that occurs with meditation, appears to be more rapidly achieved and more thorough than other indirect methods that people might use to relax—such as taking a nap, reading a book, or watching television. Part of this simply has to do with our attention: if we pay attention to something, we can do it better. If we read a book to relax, we may relax, but our mind is still paying attention to the book. The relaxation can be enhanced if we know how to pay attention to the relaxation process itself. This attentiveness is the basis for what are commonly called "relaxation techniques," such as Edmund Jacobsen's technique of "Progressive Muscular Relaxation" or Wolfgang Luthe's "Autogenic Training Program." In general, what these techniques hold in common is the focus of our attention on various parts of the body to develop an awareness of the sensations of tension or relaxation arising from these areas, coupled with an intent to relax.

There are actually two separate components to most relaxation techniques. First, the focus of attention is placed on a neutral or relaxing image, thereby removing stress-inducing thoughts from the mind. Just doing this will help interrupt the cycle of tension, and the muscles will begin to relax, especially as the flux of constantly changing thoughts begins to quiet down. Second, the process of physical relaxation can be facilitated if the focal point for our attention is the body itself, particularly the areas reflecting tension, such as within certain muscles.

It is a skill of great accomplishment to be able to maintain within the mind a single focus of attention, and this is greatly impeded by residual tensions in either the body or the psyche. In a sense, the ability to relax appears prevented by the very same factors that give rise to the need to relax. Moving one's inner awareness from point to point throughout the muscles of the body is a way to give release to the mental restlessness arising from tension without interrupting the overall process of relaxation.

Relaxation is a systematic, conscious, and comfortable process. The first step is to obtain a suitable body position for relaxation. A classic relaxation posture in yoga is known as the corpse pose, or *shavasana*. It is described below.

RELAXATION EXERCISE

Lie on the back and gently close the eyes. Place the feet a comfortable distance apart; place the arms away from the sides of the body, with the palms upward and the fingers gently curled. The legs should not touch each other, nor should the arms and hands touch the body. Do not lie haphazardly or place the limbs far apart, but lie in a symmetrical position with the head, neck, and trunk aligned.

Once a comfortable posture is achieved there are a number of relaxation procedures that can be used. The procedure given below is designed to relax the skeletal muscles, eliminate fatigue and strain, and energize both mind and body. During this exercise keep the mind alert and concentrated on the breath as the muscles are progressively relaxed. The entire exercise should require no more than ten minutes.

Lie in the corpse posture with the eyes gently closed. Inhale and exhale through the nostrils slowly, smoothly, and deeply. There should be no noise, jerks, or pauses in the breath; let the inhalations and exhalations flow naturally without exertion in one continuous movement. Keep the body still. Mentally travel through the body and relax the top of the head, forehead, eyebrows, space between the eyebrows, eyes, eyelids, cheeks, and nose. Exhale and inhale completely four times.

Relax the fingertips, fingers, hands, wrists, lower arms, upper arms, shoulders, upper back, and chest. Concentrate on the center of the chest, and exhale and inhale completely four times.

Relax the stomach, abdomen, lower back, hips, thighs, knees, calves, ankles, feet, and toes. Exhale as though your whole body is exhaling, and inhale as though your whole body is inhaling. Expel all your tension, worries, and anxieties; inhale vital energy, peace, and relaxation. Exhale and inhale completely four times.

Relax the toes, feet, ankles, calves, thighs, knees, hips, lower back, abdomen, stomach, and chest. Concentrating on the center of the chest, exhale and inhale completely four times.

Relax the upper back, shoulders, upper arms, lower arms, wrists, hands, fingers, and fingertips. Exhale and inhale completely four times.

Relax the fingertips, fingers, hands, wrists, lower arms, upper arms, shoulders, neck, chin, jaw, mouth and nostrils. Exhale and inhale completely four times.

Relax the cheeks, eyelids, eyes, eyebrows, space between the eyebrows, forehead, and the top of the head. Now, for 30 to 60 seconds, let your mind be aware of the calm and serene flow of the breath . . . let your mind make a gentle, conscious effort to guide your breath so that it remains smooth, calm, and deep, without any noise or jerks.

The most fundamental determinant of the inappropriate buildup of tension, either psychological or physical, as well as of the capacity to recover quickly, concerns the mental attitude or expectancy underlying one's activity—whether the activity be that of daily living, work, recreation, exercise, or the process of relaxation itself. If we respond to an activity with a dominant mental attitude of the achievement of a specific goal, some degree of sympathetic activation can occur whenever we face obstacles to attaining the goal. We tend to interpret an obstacle to attaining the goal, or an event that did not work out the way we planned or wished, as a threat to our ultimate success and well-being. This can be an appropriate cue to activate ourselves to try harder and thereby overcome the obstacle—unless our response is out of proportion to the need. If we carry within us the attitude that we may not achieve a desired goal, that we may fail, then small obstacles may appear larger or more significant than they really are, and our response of sympathetic activation will then be excessive.

In fact, to some degree, sympathetic activity can occur whenever we try to "do" anything, including "trying" to relax. In some persons, the attempt to relax or breathe diaphragmatically or run properly can of itself create a significant anxiety related to concern about whether one is going to perform up to expected standards—a so-called performance anxiety. All of us experience this in some measure. The question, then, is: How is it possible to relax without really trying? The way out of the dilemma takes advantage of a recurrent theme in the literature of yoga and meditation: the process of quiet observation is an "act" that need not activate any of our tension-producing reflexes. Observing our thoughts, observing the breath, observing the tension in our muscles, without trying to "do" anything—including trying to relax—will often by itself create a relaxation response automatically. The process of observing and the process of acting seem to create different physiological responses in the body—and an awareness of this can be useful in the management of stress. So an important theme in stress management needs to be "relaxation in action": how to act with the degree of relaxation—or conversely, the amount of activation—appropriate to the task.

Practice in relaxation techniques, diaphragmatic breathing, and breath awareness are important in learning how to do this, but practice in action is essential to mastery of the skill. Both aerobics and hatha yoga provide an excellent opportunity to practice the principles of relaxation and breath awareness while undertaking a physical activity. Paying attention to this dimension while exercising should result in our energy being used more efficiently, thus reducing fatigue and the risk of injury, and providing an intermediate step in acquiring relaxation skills we can use to lessen the stress of our daily activities.

We might conclude this chapter by stating that the best way to minimize tension is to prevent it from occurring in the first place. Regular practice of exercises and relaxation helps us to establish a sense of what a relaxed state is and what it feels like. This inner knowledge serves as a reference point, allowing us to notice tension as it occurs and builds up during our daily activities, and to release it. Moreover, this reference point of a relaxed feeling allows us to evaluate the manner in which we perform everyday actions. And if we have excessive tension we can use our relaxation skills to release it on a minute-to-minute basis. Soon relaxation skills provide an excellent foundation for the management of stress.

CHAPTER 3
Diet and Stress

Rudolph Ballentine, M.D.

As researchers have become more sophisticated about the subject of stress, it has become increasingly clear that what has come to be called "stress reaction" is not inherently related to what is happening around one. In other words, whether or not we respond to environmental phenomena as stressors depends to a great extent on our attitudes and on the way we see ourselves and the world around us. Thus, understanding the mind is critical to reducing stress.

There is, however, another aspect of the organism that is involved in aggravating or magnifying stress response, namely, the organism's physiological condition. Whether the organism is psychologically conditioned to view a given situation as threatening or stressful is one matter, but whether it is physically and physiologically capable of dealing with the situation is another matter entirely—and one that may also greatly contribute to the development of the crisis.

This distinction is like that made between the software and hardware of a computer. Software has to do with how

Reprinted from Dawn *magazine, Vol. 2, Number 2, 1982*

the computer is programmed and how it processes information. Hardware, on the other hand, has to do with the physical condition of the machine, such as how many circuits it has, what kind of currents they can carry, and whether or not the machine has the capacity to handle certain kinds of input.

In a similar way, the human subject may have re-educated himself to the point of being better able to deal psychologically with environmental situations or stressors, but if his metabolism and nervous system are unhealthy and functioning poorly, he may still be easily shaken by relatively modest demands. It is here—in the area of maintaining the body in optimal condition and keeping the physiological machinery in good order so it can respond accurately, flexibly, and comfortably—that nutrition plays such an important part.

The first and probably simplest point here is the scheduling of meals. Whether or not we have recently eaten may determine to what extent we are able to deal successfully with stress. Entering a conference room immediately after a large heavy meal is certainly one of the most frequently made mistakes by overworked executives.

Our systems are designed in such a way that metabolism can be geared in one of two ways: either it can be dedicated to digestion and assimilation of food and to the processes of cleansing that are the work of the bowels, kidneys, liver, and so forth, or it can be directed toward dealing with the external environment. Thus, whenever we have to deal with external stimuli while our bodies are geared toward digesting food, there is a serious and uncomfortable internal conflict. During digestion, blood is diverted to the digestive tract away from the brain, and our ability to think clearly is seriously impaired. Words won't come out; thoughts are processed poorly.

In a very stressful situation this may be enough to tip the balance toward serious decompensation: we begin to feel anxious, nervous, and upset, and find that we simply can't handle the situation. The timing of meals is, therefore, extremely important. While this is a relatively simple and commonsensical issue, it is overlooked surprisingly often. When he should schedule his meals simply doesn't enter the average person's mind as he plans challenging or demanding work.

Overeating is a related phenomenon. Eating a very large meal, especially one that is oily or greasy, will tend to delay the digestive process. Such a meal can preoccupy the body's metabolism and blood flow for many hours afterwards. Improperly chewing food can also, of course, delay its digestion. In either case, clarity and quickness of mind are impaired for a long time after eating.

The extent to which one's mind is clear can be related to other aspects of the diet, too. For example, foods extremely high in protein or extremely high in fats and oils require increased excretion on the part of the liver and kidneys. In other words, this means that it takes some extra work and time for the organs of elimination to clear the blood of the substances that result from protein and fat digestion. Until these wastes are cleared from the blood there will be some impairment of consciousness and lack of clarity in the mind. For example, one who has cultivated some degree of self-awareness will find that a meal of fried potatoes, oily dressings, and tempura will leave him feeling clouded and murky. Blood oil and fat levels go up just after such a meal; later on, so do the metabolites of such oils and fats. During all this time, logical thinking and decision making are hindered. While this may be relatively minor in most cases, it can be an added burden that tends to tip the scales toward reacting in a stressed way to demands and situations around us.

Highly processed foods often contain a smaller percentage of intact nutrients than do whole foods. In other words, many of the molecules in processed foods have been damaged or destroyed through the heating, chemical treatment, or other processes through which the food has gone. These damaged molecules, if no longer useful as nutrients, further contribute to the excretory burden with which the body must cope. Here again we are overtaxing the organs of elimination and producing a situation in which the nervous system is exposed to blood that has not been entirely or optimally cleared of those metabolic by-products that might interfere with its functioning. This is true not only of processed foods but also of those foods that have been improperly cooked—that are oversalted, cooked too long, or prepared in combinations that make digestion difficult. Even undercooked food can prolong digestion or cause it to be incomplete so that undesirable by-products are released into the blood.

Fuel delivery is the next important area in which nutrition and eating habits may greatly influence the capacity of the organism to deal with stress. By "fuel" is meant primarily carbohydrate, since it is glucose that is mainly responsible for the energy on which the body runs. Glucose enters the blood as a result of the conversion of sugar or starch; it is then carried to the tissues where it enters the cells to supply energy. This is the basic source of energy for all the body, including the nervous system. If the blood sugar level drops below a certain level, then the supply of fuel for the nervous system itself is jeopardized. At that point a person will begin to feel nervous, irritable, shaky, and hard-pressed to deal with the most ordinary demands from the environment. For this reason, maintaining adequate and well-modulated blood sugar levels is one of the priorities of the body's design.

Blood sugar is to a great extent regulated by the secretion of insulin, since insulin allows glucose to move from the bloodstream to the cells. In diabetics, who have a shortage of internally produced insulin, if the condition becomes severe, blood sugar levels may drop to the point that glucose no longer reaches the brain cells. There is then a loss of consciousness, called a diabetic coma.

In a healthy person, or even in a diabetic who properly administers insulin to the cells, such a severe condition is not likely to occur. However, milder versions of the same thing can happen if the blood sugar level drops below a certain point. Low blood sugar is called "hypoglycemia" (*hypo* means low; *glycemia* refers to the level of sugar in the blood). In many people, fluctuations in blood sugar are produced primarily by dietary habits, particularly by taking in concentrated sugar.

Glucose resulting from the breakdown of starch is produced slowly as the starch is being digested. Sugar, on the other hand, rushes into the bloodstream wholesale, as it were, causing the blood glucose level to shoot up rapidly. Such an experience is sometimes called a "sugar high," and is often sought after by those who are weak and exhausted. The response of the body, however, is to secrete a large dose of insulin into the bloodstream in an attempt to move the sugar out of the blood and into the cells so as to bring the blood sugar back down to normal level. The body did not evolve around the use of concentrated sugar in the diet and is basically ill-equipped to deal with it. Therefore the drastic insulin response marshaled to deal with the excess input of sugar results in an equally drastic drop in blood sugar. Frequently this is so severe that the functioning of the nervous system is impaired. In other words, if you eat a couple of candy bars on an empty stomach, you are likely to feel an initial surge of energy but a subsequent irritability and perhaps anxiety with a reduced capability to cope with stress. The entire unfortunate sequence of events is due to a poorly regulated input of fuel. In this case it might be useful to think of the body and the nervous system functioning as a machine. If it does not get an adequate and consistent supply of fuel, then its performance will be unsatisfactory.

Similar up and down cycles can be initiated by stimulants such as caffeine. Again there is an initial phase during which one feels a sense of increased energy and a subsequent phase of a sort of rebound effect or excessive fatigue. Sugar and caffeine are only the most obvious of the quick-energy fixes to which we resort. Salt is also a stimulant. One of the reasons many people have difficulty reducing salt in the diet is that without salt they feel a sense of tiredness. This is due to a loss of the stimulation that had come from the salt, as well as increased difficulty in digesting foods without this stimulant. Even concentrated protein can act as a stimulant, and the washed-out, letdown feeling that results when large amounts of eggs, cheese, and so forth are omitted from the diet is partly due to this. Using foods as stimulants can sometimes be managed quite capably, but if one stimulant piles on top of another in a frantic attempt to artificially sustain activity and replace rest, then a person is setting up a metabolic booby trap for himself and will eventually be done in by it.

There is one more major problem that frequently and seriously impairs the capacity of the organism to respond to stress, namely, a deficiency of vitamins or minerals. Though we often hear the (probably accurate) comment that Americans take many unnecessary supplements, deficiencies of vitamins and minerals still play a considerable role in health and stress problems. To understand why this is so, it is necessary to look at the role played by vitamins and minerals in the metabolic functioning of the body.

We might say that all vital processes of the cells (and this includes the cells of the nervous system) are formed by a multiplicity of biochemical reactions. Each reaction may be looked at individually, and many of them can be duplicated in a test tube. On the whole, however, outside the body these chemical reactions proceed much too slowly to sustain life. In the protoplasm of the cell, they must move rapidly so that the functions of the body can be carried out at a rate that is in keeping with the demands of the environment. The increased rapidity of chemical reactions of the body is made possible by the functioning of special catalysts that encourage and facilitate the interactions of the molecules. These catalysts, called enzymes, are huge proteins specialized for this purpose.

The enzyme is designed in such a way that the molecules that must react with it fit into it like a key fits into a lock. Two molecules that are to join together (or a large molecule that is to be split) are brought by the enzymes into contact with a single critical atom located at the exact site of the chemical reaction. This single atom at the business end of the enzyme molecule is always a mineral such as zinc, chromium, or copper. This huge enzyme molecule requires only one single atom of the metal in question. These minerals, which are so very crucial to body functioning, are found in the body's tissues in only the most minute quantities. For this reason they are often called trace minerals. For many years they were considered by biologists as unrelated to metabolic processes and were thought to be present only as incidental contaminants.

In recent years we have discovered increasingly the importance of these trace minerals, and it appears that we still have not identified all of the minerals that play important roles in the body's metabolism. For example, recently it has been discovered that arsenic, while toxic in large amounts, is in minute quantities absolutely essential to life. A moment's reflection makes it obvious why the trace minerals are so critical to bodily functions and to the ability to cope with external demands: every step of tissue functioning is dependent on the proper and timely occurrence of metabolic reactions, and every metabolic reaction is in turn dependent on the presence of adequate enzymes to facilitate it. In turn, however, the manufacture of enzymes is dependent on adequate supplies of trace minerals, and although only tiny amounts are needed, even such small quantities are often not available in the foodstuffs that nowadays are commonly consumed in the United States.

Highly processed foods, such as packaged snacks, white flour, and white sugar, have been largely depleted of their trace mineral content. They bring calories, they can supply the glucose that is needed for the body's fuel supplies, but they are unable to supply the trace minerals necessary for the metabolic machinery that will burn the glucose. The situation that results is much like an automobile that has plenty of gas but no spark plugs. It simply won't go. It is not uncommon to find people who complain that though they feel hungry and eat a lot they still have no energy. They feel tired and simply don't feel up to the challenges that confront them.

White sugar and white flour are notorious examples of what are commonly called stripped calories, or empty calories; that is, they contain the carbohydrates needed for a fuel supply but they do not bring with them the where-withal to burn the fuel. The American diet has been criticized for containing large quantities of empty carbo-hydrates. Twenty to twenty-five percent of the calories in the average American diet comes from added sweeteners, such as sugar and corn syrup.

This is, however, only a minor problem when com-pared to the consumption of fats and oils. Fats and oils are also primarily empty carbohydrates, devoid of any nutri-tion other than the ability to supply fuel. They can be burned (albeit with some difficulty) to supply energy, but they bring with them no minerals and virtually no vita-mins. While sugar may be twenty to twenty-five percent of the calories in the American diet, fats and oils constitute forty to forty-five percent. The sheer magnitude of such an intake of fats and oils is shocking. Small wonder that the American diet is often characterized as "greasy." There are few population groups in the world that consume more fats and oils than do the inhabitants of the U.S.A.

The total, then, of fat, oil, and sugar in the diet will range on the average between sixty and seventy percent. This means that only thirty to forty percent of the diet brings with it the vitamins and minerals needed for proper metabolism. Actually, even that thirty to forty percent of the diet, if it is of poor quality, may not bring with it the required nutrients for its own use. Such foods as white bread, canned vegetables, and instant mashed potatoes contain too few vitamins and minerals for even their own processing. By contrast, whole foods—such as whole grains, beans, fresh vegetables, and fruit—bring with them a full complement of the micronutrients (vitamins and minerals) that are necessary in the burning of the glucose that they contain. This is why it is so important to stress the use of whole foods for good health and for the ability to deal with stress.

Much as minerals contribute to the manufacture of enzymes, vitamins are also often components of enzyme molecules the body cannot manufacture, which must be taken in the diet preformed. In a typical American diet, the vitamin intake will often be sub-optimal, whereas environmental stressors may be very frequent and severe. There are certain vitamins—vitamin C and the B complex, particularly pantothenic acid—that are especially prone to be used up in large quantities when one responds to the environment in a stressed fashion. For this reason products called "stress supplements," which include these key nutrients, are now available.

If a person wishes to modify his diet so that his dietary habit patterns might contribute to a successful program of stress management, he should consider the following points: (1) Limit processed foods; try to substitute whole, natural, fresh foods as much as possible; (2) Cut down on red meat, hard cheese, vegetable oils, salad dressing, and other oily and greasy components of the diet that contribute unduly large quantities of empty calories; (3) Try to take most carbohydrates in a complex form (that is, starch) rather than in the form of sugar, which is released too quickly in the bloodstream and disturbs the regulation of glucose levels and the proper delivery of fuel itself; and (4) Pay some attention to variations in stress levels and, when necessary, supplement the diet with appropriate vitamins.

Mineral levels in the diet can be increased by taking easily digestible mineral-rich foods. This includes well-cooked fresh vegetables, especially the leafy ones. Vegetables become an especially rich source of minerals when they have been cooked down to the point that they are both concentrated and easy to digest. Fresh vegetable juices are another source of easily assimilated mineral-rich nutrition. Mineral supplementation through tablets is, on the other hand, a difficult matter. The use of such inorganic minerals may be difficult for the body to regulate since they compete with one another for absorption, and, unless carefully prescribed, their use may aggravate or even create an imbalance of trace minerals in the body.

As an experiment, a person who wishes to study the effects of diet on stress levels might make a few simple alterations for a period of ten days and then attempt to judge the effects on his sense of well-being. The following changes would be a good starting point: (1) Eliminate all junk and fast foods; (2) Reduce sugar, white flour, and red meat; (3) Add one fresh, cooked, green (part leafy) vegetable per day; (4) Take two pieces of fresh fruit a day; (5) Take one serving of whole grains a day; and (6) Twice a day have some combination of whole grains and legumes (beans or peas). This grain/legume combination increases vegetable protein and helps replace protein lost by reducing meat intake. Drastic changes should never be made in the diet, and these modifications should be made in a gradual way. In other words, reducing meat does not mean eliminating it completely if one has been on a very high meat diet. If moderate changes are made and sustained for a ten-day period, one should experience noticeable benefits. It is very important to remember that dietary changes should not be made mechanically. Following a printed diet rigidly will only lead to discouragement and distaste. The basic strategy for successfully improving one's diet is to learn to gear dietary intake to nutritional needs. This can be accomplished only by cultivating an increased level of self-awareness. One must learn to become sensitive to the signals from within oneself that offer cues as to what is needed and when. How much to eat, when to eat it, which foods to eat today, which foods to eat tomorrow, can only be judged by learning to read what the body is saying. In other words, ultimately the regulation of diet hinges on the same issue as does the regulation of psychological processes. Attitudes, ways of thinking, and perception influence one's psychological stance and set the stage for experiencing the world as stressful, just as debility of the body and nervous system from poor nutrition undermines one's ability to respond comfortably, flexibly, and adaptively.

In both of these areas—physiological well-being and psychological predisposition—one's potential for reducing the tendency to stress reactions will hinge on increasing one's level of self-awareness, learning to study oneself and one's needs, and attuning oneself to internal signals so as to be able to make the proper modifications in expectations, behavior, diet, breathing, and relaxation. Skillful use of both body and mind enables one to become dynamic and creative and to progressively free oneself from the susceptibility to suffer from stress.

CHAPTER 4
Breath: The Way of Balance

Phil Nuernberger, Ph.D.

One of the most important skills for managing stress is learning to regulate the breath. Modern clinicians and researchers are increasingly discovering the important role that breath can play in overcoming mental and physical tension, while in the ancient traditions of self-development, harmonizing the breath has always been seen as a gateway to inner work. The following parable from the East may help to underscore the importance of breath.

Once upon a time there was a great gathering of all the active and passive senses of man for the purpose of deciding which of them was to be king. They were all dressed in their finest, most impressive clothing, and each was busily trying to impress the others with its importance and power. The sense of sight was dressed in shimmering, brilliant colors and spoke movingly of the utility and beauty of his power. The sense of sound, garbed in subtle clothing that moved and sounded like a gentle wind in the trees, and wearing jewelry that tinkled like tiny, clear silver bells, argued just as movingly for his power. All the others, each beautifully robed, were as loud and insistent, each attempting to outshine the others.

Reprinted from Dawn *magazine, Vol. 2, Number 2, 1982*

Finally, breath, unnoticed in his common and ordinary clothing, tired of the useless noise and senseless argument, announced in a strong voice that the decision was already made, and that he, the breath, was the most vital, and thus king of all. There was a stunned silence, and then a clamoring racket of denial and argument as each pointed out its own beauty and power. Having heard enough, and somewhat irritated by all the hubbub and foolishness, breath decided to leave, and almost as unnoticed as when he was there, he quietly slipped out the door. Within a few moments, all the other senses began to dim, and their power and beauty began to fade. Finally realizing the power of breath, all the other senses called after him and begged his return, paying full respect to his sovereignty.

This ancient yogic story about the importance of breath is still very relevant to our modern Western society. In our fast-paced, exciting, technological society, we become attracted to and charmed by the sensory experiences of life. We become hypnotized by and addicted to the changes, sensory stimulation, and distractions that are so available (even unavoidable) to Western ears. In a very real sense we lose awareness of the fundamental realities within ourselves and become unconscious of the various harmonies, levels, and processes that constitute the inner reality. We thus lose awareness of the inherent harmony and joy of life itself. As a consequence, we have become subject to the whims of our senses, and have become the source of our own discomfort, disease, and suffering. Nowhere is this more apparent than in the critical problem of stress and its consequences, which plague many of us on a daily basis. And it is here that the breath, unnoticed because it is unlooked for, plays its vital role.

In Western society, where medicine and psychology are grounded in a primitive Newtonian materialism, stress is understood in the framework of physiological reductionism and has come to be seen as a technological problem of symptom removal: something is wrong with the body or with the behavior, so it obviously must be fixed. In order to remove the symptom and thus fix the body, simply add the right chemical (medication), repair or remove the "broken part" (just as with any good machine), or manipulate the environmental "reinforcers" (in other words, change the office, the home, the society, the world!) that "control" the behavior, and attempt to condition more "proper" behavior (which means behavior that is more useful, correct, desired, socially adaptive, or socially approved).

This represents a good, solid, "scientific," and technological method, and characterizes the Western approach to stress and, consequently, stress management. Relaxation exercises, often done to music and soft lights or with the accompaniment of sophisticated biofeedback equipment, are most often simply an extension of this materialistic "technological fix" approach. The main difficulty with this approach is that it doesn't work very well. Symptom removal doesn't alter causal factors, and relaxation exercises don't eliminate stress. In fact, the current Western approach to stress is riddled with illogical statements such as, "stress is both good and bad for you." It also includes meaningless definitions such as, "Stress is the body's nonspecific response to stimuli"—a definition akin to saying that you are alive and being alive is stressful, and is burdened by an excess baggage of professional jargon, such as "eustress" (good stress) and distress (bad stress)—concerning which no one can tell the difference except that the consequence of one is that you feel fine and the consequence of the other is that you keel over with a heart attack. How to recognize one from the other before the consequence manifests seems to be left to the individual, as participant in a game of stress roulette. For the loser, we have marvelously sophisticated Intensive Care Units. The winner, of course, gets to continue to play the game.

The truth is that this mechanistic approach, with all of its technological sophistication and excitement, is pretty much a dismal failure. The American public is not becoming healthier. The incidence of chronic disease has continued to increase every year. Nor do we seem any happier or more successful in our personal lives: divorce has reached the fifty percent level; alcoholism affects ten percent of the work force; one of every six Americans is on a major tranquilizer.

What has begun to work is a holistic approach to stress that incorporates a perspective which includes all levels of human functioning—not just the physical, behavioral, or environmental. What has begun to lead individuals to health and happiness is the development of self-responsibility built on a firm foundation of self-knowledge, self-regulation, and self-discipline. The most complete science to provide that foundation is yoga, a holistic science of human functioning at all capacities and levels that includes the practical understanding and techniques which lead to self-regulation through increasing self-awareness.

In yoga science, human functioning is understood as a complex harmonization of different levels of energy. This energy, called *prana,* ranges from very subtle (*sattvic*) manifestations such as is found in the most subtle aspect of mind—the discriminative aspect, called *buddhi*—to the most dense (*tamasic*) form of bound energy, represented by the material expression of the body and its physiological processes. It is this profound knowledge of energy structures and patterns that provides a logical framework for understanding stress, or dysfunction, and leads directly to the ability to regulate stress and eventually become free from its consequences.

From a yogic perspective, we can understand stress to be an imbalance or disharmony within and between the various levels of human functioning. At the physical level (referred to in yoga as the *annamaya kosha,* or food sheath), this disharmony is characterized by an imbalance within the autonomic nervous system. The autonomic nervous system is actually composed of two anatomically distinct nervous systems: the sympathetic system, which regulates excitation; and the parasympathetic, which regulates inhibition. These two systems are designed to work in harmony with each other. When this balance or harmony is disturbed, we then have a condition of stress. In other words, stress means that we are physiologically out of balance. The fact that we have either arousal or inhibition does not, in and of itself, mean that we have stress. The key element in defining the physiological parameters of stress is whether or not there exists a balance, either dynamically or as a total harmonization, between sympathetic and parasympathetic activity. Autonomic imbalance is stress.

Autonomic balance is best understood as a dynamic harmonization of neurological activity, leading to balanced functioning of other physiological systems. If we understand stress as an imbalance, characterized on one hand as "fight or flight" (arousal) and on the other hand as the "possum response" (inhibition), our entire approach to stress is reformulated in such a way as to lead to the yogic understanding of the mind/body relationship and to very powerful tools for self-regulation and control.

Traditionally, Western science has denied the possibility of direct or conscious regulation of autonomic functioning. This denial is based on limited experience and is a direct consequence of biological and behavioral reductionism. (Remember the high school health class where the teacher would read directly out of the book and state categorically, "You cannot control certain parts or functions of the body"? Did it ever make you wonder just who did control the body?) In yoga science, however, autonomic functioning is understood not only in relation to other physiological structures (such as the limbic system in

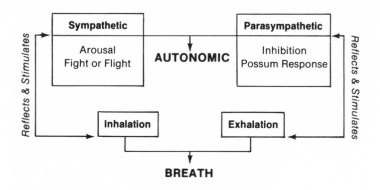

Figure 1
Breath and Autonomic Balance
Source: Nuernberger: *Freedom from Stress: A Holistic Approach*

the brain) but also in relation to the underlying energy structures that form the basis for the physical event (process or structure). The immediate underlying level to the physical body (annamaya kosha) is called the *pranamaya kosha,* or energy sheath. Within this subtle level, we find that the major vehicle for the exchange and regulation of energy (prana) is the breath.

According to yoga science, autonomic functioning can be directly regulated by the breath. At the physical level, where energy manifests itself in one way through neural activity, there is a subtle but direct relationship between autonomic activity and breathing. As shown in the accompanying figure, the inhalation reflects and stimulates sympathetic discharge, while the exhalation reflects and stimulates parasympathetic discharge. If the breath is disturbed, then autonomic balance is disturbed, and there is a condition of stress. If the autonomic balance becomes disturbed (for example, from fearful thoughts or a poor diet), then the breath will reflect this disturbance and flow irregularly.

On the other hand, proper regulation of the breath can

reestablish autonomic balance and resolve the stress. The reestablishment of proper breathing habits allows us to develop our capacity to regulate the autonomic nervous system consciously and directly—a critical and necessary step in the self-regulation of stress. While it may seem surprising that such a common, generally unnoticed activity as respiration has such power, our language reflects an unconscious awareness of this relationship between autonomic activity and the breath. To illustrate: if there is an attack to the body, resulting in a sharp pain, there is an immediate and strong response of the sympathetic "fight or flight" alarm system resulting in instant arousal and mobilization of the body's resources. What then happens to the breath? There is a sharp inhalation: we "gasp with pain." In contrast to this, have you ever heard of anyone speak of a "gasp of depression"? Of course not; instead, what is always heard is a reference to "sighs of depression," reflecting the strong parasympathetic dominance that characterizes depression.

On a more subtle level of functioning, there is an emerging awareness of a critical relationship between breathing and cardiovascular functioning. Knowledgeable cardiologists now feel that breathing can critically influence cardiovascular functioning in at least four ways. Probably the most critical relationship is the effect of breathing on the electrical activity of the heart. Autonomic tone regulates the subtle exchange of potassium and sodium ions in the pacemaker cells of the heart in the sino-atrial node. This exchange is what determines the actual beating of the heart. The action of the breath, particularly in terms of respiratory motion, in regulating autonomic tone can directly influence this electrical activity of the heart. This influence can be so important that at least one researcher states that those who suffer heart attack due to arrhythmia can really be said to have more of a breathing problem than a heart problem.

In other words, the way we breathe can lead to direct interference with the electrical activity of the heart. One example of a deadly breathing pattern is the sustained and regular pattern of apnea, the involuntary retention of breath commonly found in heart patients. It is also found, unfortunately, in a large percentage of the general public.

Breathing also influences blood pressure in at least three ways. The way we breathe influences how much blood enters the heart, which is called "pre-load." This directly affects the force with which the heart must pump the blood out, and thus is a major factor in determining blood pressure. The way we breathe also determines the quality of the blood in terms of the level of carbonic acid (carbon dioxide). Through improper breathing, levels of carbon dioxide are allowed to remain high, adversely affecting blood gases and, in turn, blood pressure. If we breathe in such a way as to create a state of arousal, this sympathetic action begins to constrict peripheral blood vessels and can lead directly to an elevation of blood pressure. These mechanisms and the effect of breathing are explored in greater detail in Chapter 9 of this book, in the article titled, "Stress, A New. Perspective."

What all this means, of course, is that breathing—an activity we all do and generally pay very little attention to—is quite probably the single most important tool in stress management. Unfortunately, most individuals in American society breathe in such a way as to create imbalance, rather than in a way that will lead to and maintain proper balance. In other words, most of us have poor breathing patterns that create stress and disturb us both physically and emotionally.

Some of these poor breathing habits are shallow breathing; irregular breathing with uneven inhalation/exhalation cycles; frequent pauses, or stopping (holding) the flow of breath; mouth breathing; and (most common) a dependence on chest breathing (more correctly called thoracic breathing), which is nothing more than a bad habit conditioned by years of tight clothing, poor posture, cultural influences, and emotional shocks. From the author's experience, roughly ninety percent of the American public breathes in such a way as to create and maintain stress.

The good news, however, is that with a little consistent effort, breathing patterns can be established that will bring balance back to the body and help regulate emotions. The basic task is to reestablish diaphragmatic-dominated breathing as the moment-to-moment respiratory pattern. Diaphragmatic breathing is the body's natural method and provides a harmonizing effect on the autonomic system as well as allowing the most efficient gas exchange within the lungs. Breathing provides both a nourishing and a cleansing function for the body. The oxygen brought in with the inhalation is utilized by every cell of the body. When the gas exchange (oxygen entering the blood and carbon dioxide being cleansed from the blood) is not done efficiently— such as occurs during chest breathing dominance—then the entire pulmonary-cardiovascular system must work harder in order to supply the proper oxygenation to the blood.

Just as important is the cleansing action, the removal from the blood of carbon dioxide, a waste product that can create problems if not properly removed. Again, chest breathing does not cleanse the lungs as completely as diaphragmatic breathing, thus allowing the blood gases to be more acidic. The importance of diaphragmatic breathing, then, is due in large measure to the increased efficiency of getting oxygen into the blood and of removing the carbon dioxide. Diaphragmatic breathing also requires much less muscular effort than chest breathing, and thus does not utilize as much energy. Those who reestablish diaphragmatic breathing as their moment-to-moment breathing pattern will find that they are not as tired at the end of the day, simply because of the increased efficiency and the decreased energy expenditure.

Chest breathing is directly associated with sympathetic arousal in the body. Consequently, when breathing with the chest, you are really signaling your body: "Get prepared, there is something you need to protect yourself from!" This can be so drastic that many individuals suffer from anxiety attacks simply because of poor breathing habits; that is, they breathe primarily with their chest, and this precipitates the anxiety attack. The common psychiatric label for this is "free-floating anxiety," and is rarely recognized to be a breathing problem. By retraining the breathing habits and developing moment-to-moment diaphragmatic breathing instead of chest breathing, very often the anxiety states completely disappear.

Also of importance is respiratory motion, which must be even and steady if balance is to be achieved. Irregular, jerky breaths that are not balanced between inhalation and exhalation will lead directly to autonomic imbalance. Pauses in the breath not only reflect apnea (and possibly create pressure on the cardiovascular system) but also disturb the entire autonomic balance. In deep concentration, the breath will become very quiet, and often so slight that it is hard to tell if the person is breathing. This is a natural consequence of deep concentration and its effect on the body. However, most people have pauses and jerks due not to concentration but to poor breathing habits, and these wreak havoc on the nervous system. Consistent practice of smooth, even breathing will result in a greater control over respiratory motion and lead to a state of mental and physical calmness and alertness. Of course a smooth, even motion depends on diaphragmatic control and is very difficult to achieve when one is a chest breather.

In practical terms, the breath is a very powerful tool in the regulation of stress and, consequently, in altering the symptoms associated with stress. In yoga science, where regulation of the breath plays a central role in pranayama (the control of prana, or energy), there are a great number of breathing exercises. A few are given below. These can be practiced easily and safely by the beginner, and are basic to any attempt to control stress.

As critical as proper breathing is in the regulation of stress, it is only a powerful mediating factor, and does not have direct control over the autonomic nervous system. In the structure of the nervous system, the autonomic system (part of the peripheral nervous system), is under the direct control of the central nervous system, and in particular of the limbic system. The limbic system is a part of the brain that is responsible for the so-called "vegetative functions" of the body, such as regulation of arterial pressure, body fluid balance, electrolyte content of body fluids, gastrointestinal activity, and many internal secretions of the endocrine glands. The limbic system is also responsible for much of the emotional response in man, and is often referred to as the "seat of the emotions."

The limbic system, however, is in turn regulated by the "highest" brain center, the cerebral cortex. It is here that the "intellectual" activities occur: the thoughts, images, memories, perceptual integrations, and interpretations. According to the decisions made in the cortex, the limbic system is activated, and then all the endocrine glands and the autonomic nervous system are activated. Thus ultimately it is our mind that determines whether or not we suffer from stress. The cerebral cortex is the control room of the mind. Stress is a clear example of a mental and physiological process, or mind/body interaction.

In yoga science, the relationship between mind and body is understood to be mediated by energy (prana), and the laws governing this relationship are well known. Here again, breath—as the major vehicle for prana—plays a significant role. In many vital ways, the breath represents and reflects this relationship between mind and body. This is the most obvious in the interaction between the mind and the autonomic nervous system. While the mind has the power to control the body, it is, in turn, influenced by events in the body. Even in Western psychology, it is well known that mental anxiety is not possible if the individual is relaxed. By maintaining an even, steady breath, a state of physiological balance is maintained, allowing the mind to remain balanced. Thus, a significant degree of control over the emotions can be achieved when one is able to regulate the breath.

On a more subtle level, awareness of the breath can lead to control over the actual events within the stream of consciousness itself. This is surprisingly simple and direct. Most of us are fairly locked into one aspect of our mental processes: the thinking process. This manifests itself in an almost constant chatter within the mind. Left uncontrolled, this chatter is a great source of stress for the individual, as the mind constantly jumps from past to future with little focus on the here and now. This problem-solving aspect of looking within mind, if not focused on an immediate problem in the environment, will create a problem to solve in the mind. This is done through anticipation, and is the basis for fear, which thus triggers the alarm responses.

By bringing the focus of attention to the *feeling* of the breath as it enters the nostrils, an individual is able to stop this chatter immediately. The mind becomes clear, and the inner chatter stops. In more psychological terms, the individual moves from a cognizing, abstracting mode of being to a more pristine, perceptual mode of being. In other words, we stop talking to ourselves and start being more aware of the world around us. This simple technique of breath awareness gradually leads one to a greater degree of control over his thoughts and to a greater sensitivity to both internal and external events. Consequently, one is able to act and respond more effectively in the world.

So it is that the breath, which supplies us with the vital energy that sustains our life, is also the very tool that can lead us to a more joyful experience of that life. Patient study and training of the breath is necessary if we are to be free from the imbalance we call stress. It is within our power. We have what we need; we simply have to become aware of that power and to use it for our benefit.

BREATHING EXERCISES

There are a number of breathing exercises that can be safely practiced by anyone. They are quite simple, and yield many benefits, and are an important part of any effective stress management program. Listed below are several breathing exercises and a sleep exercise which will alleviate insomnia. The reader is encouraged to experiment with these exercises and observe their results.

Diaphragmatic Breathing

The purpose of this exercise is to reestablish diaphragmatic breathing as the normal, everyday moment-to-moment resting breathing habit. If one does no other exercise, he should be sure to practice this one; it is that important. It will be most effective if practiced at least three times a day for ten to fifteen minutes each time; eventually, the easy rhythmic breathing will begin to replace the strained, unnatural chest breathing to which you have become habituated. Being aware of your breathing as much as possible will speed the process of change from chest breathing to diaphragmatic breathing.

To Practice: Before going to sleep and just after waking, place your right hand on your upper abdomen, with the little finger directly above the navel and the fingers spread so that the thumb is almost touching the chest. Place the left hand on the upper chest with the little finger between the two breasts. As you breathe, concentrate on the air moving down into the upper abdomen (as if you are filling your stomach with breath). The right hand should rise with the inhalation and fall with the exhalation; the left hand should not move. You should feel a slight motion in the lower portion of the chest cavity, but the upper portion should remain still. Within a few moments you will become more rested and quiet. Do not try to force the breath. Allow the motion to be gentle and effortless. Notice how easy it is to breathe deeply and easily, without any effort.

Benefits: This will lead to autonomic balance and a relaxed state, generally. After some weeks, depending on the individual, you will begin to notice subtle and gradual changes in your daily breathing patterns. Its movement will be more relaxed and rhythmic. As was discussed earlier, this leads to a greater efficiency of the pulmonary process and reduces the amount of work required for proper ventilation perfusion.

Even Breathing

While you are practicing diaphragmatic breathing, concentrate on making the breath very smooth and even. The inhalation and exhalation should be of the same length and have the same pressure. Do not exhale all the breath at the beginning of the exhalation. Concentrate on keeping the flow pressure even throughout the entire cycle. Eliminate all pauses, stops, and shakiness in the breath, including the pause between inhalation and exhalation. Imagine that the breath is like a large wheel moving through the body without any pauses or stops. It is often helpful to picture the breath flow as a completely smooth, even sine wave.

Benefits: The jerkier the breath, the more disruptive it is to the autonomic nervous system. When the breath is smooth and even, autonomic balance is achieved.

2:1 Breathing

After gaining control of diaphragmatic movement and establishing a smooth, even, rhythmic respiration, gently slow down the rate of exhalation until you are breathing out for about twice as long as you are inhaling. (It might be necessary to shorten the length of inhalation very slightly.)

You are simply changing the rhythm of the breath. You are not trying to fill the lungs completely nor empty them completely. You are only altering the motion of the lungs in a very systematic way. You may count six on the exhalation and three on the inhalation, or eight on the exhalation and four on the inhalation—or whatever is most comfortable for you. Then, after you have established this gentle rhythm, stop the mental counting and focus on the smoothness and evenness of the breath flow. Eliminate all jerks and pauses. Maintain 2:1 diaphragmatic breathing for as long as you wish.

Benefits: 2:1 breathing establishes a relaxed state in the body by very subtly stimulating the parasympathetic system more than the sympathetic system. This leads to relaxation and reduces arousal in the body even if you do it only a few moments.

The Complete Breath

In this exercise all three mechanisms of inhalation—diaphragmatic, thoracic and clavicular (collarbones)—are brought into use. Inhale first, using the diaphragm and expanding the belly; then continue the inhalation by expanding the chest; then let the inhalation continue to the very top of the lungs, at which point a slight upward movement of the clavicles may be experienced. The exhalation is done in reverse motion, letting the clavicles drop slightly, then letting the chest wall collapse slightly, then letting the belly collapse as the diaphragm moves upward, pushing the air out of the lungs. The breath should be slow and smooth, without any pauses or jerks.

This complete breath is a very useful technique to use when you are sitting at your desk and feel a lot of tension in your shoulders. A five-minute practice will be very helpful in reducing not only muscle tension but also mental fatigue.

Alternate Nostril Breathing

There are many breathing exercises, each for a specific purpose. Alternate nostril breathing is a simple exercise that purifies and balances the nervous system. Ideally this exercise should be practiced at least twice a day, in the morning and evening, doing three cycles each time. Morning and evening are the best times for regular practice, although you can practice anytime you want to calm the nervous system and clear the mind. To perform this exercise you will first need to identify your active and passive nostrils.

Usually the breath does not flow equally in both nostrils; one nostril is more congested than the other. This can be easily observed: gently close one nostril and inhale and exhale rapidly through the open nostril; then repeat the process on the opposite side. You will find that one nostril flows more freely than the other; this one is the active nostril, the other is the passive nostril. Throughout the day and night the active and passive nostrils alternate. Once you have established the active and passive nostrils, you are ready to begin the practice of alternate nostril breathing.

A. Sit in an easy and steady posture with the head, neck, and trunk straight. Inhalation and exhalation should be of equal duration. Do not force the breath; keep it slow, controlled, and free from sounds and jerks. With practice, gradually lengthen the duration of the inhalation and the exhalation.

B. Bring the right hand to the nose, folding the index finger and the middle finger so that the right thumb can be used to close the right nostril and the ring finger can be used to close the left nostril.

C. Close the passive nostril and exhale completely through the active nostril.

D. At the end of the exhalation, close the active nostril

and inhale through the passive nostril slowly and completely. Inhalation and exhalation should be of equal duration.

E. Repeat this cycle of exhalation with the active nostril and inhalation with the passive nostril two more times.

F. At the end of the third inhalation with the passive nostril, exhale completely through the same nostril, keeping the active nostril closed with the finger or thumb.

G. At the end of the exhalation, close the passive nostril and inhale through the active nostril.

H. Repeat two more times the cycle of exhalation through the passive nostril and inhalation through the active nostril.

To sum up:

1.	Exhale	Active
2.	Inhale	Passive
3.	Exhale	Active
4.	Inhale	Passive
5.	Exhale	Active
6.	Inhale	Passive
7.	Exhale	Passive
8.	Inhale	Active
9.	Exhale	Passive
10.	Inhale	Active
11.	Exhale	Passive
12.	Inhale	Active

J. Place the hands on the knees and exhale and inhale through both nostrils evenly for three complete breaths. This completes ONE cycle of alternate nostril breathing. Perform two more cycles.

Sleep Exercise

Breathing is a key element in relaxation, and this exercise uses your breathing process to help you get to sleep. It will also help you sleep more restfully. The following steps make up the exercise. Follow them closely:

All breathing is done at the ratio of 2:1. Exhale for twice as long as you inhale. Use a comfortable count such as 6:3 or 8:4. You are not trying to completely empty or fill the lungs. The 2:1 ratio should be effortless. Pay close attention to your breath. There should be no stops, pauses, or shakiness during either the inhalation or the exhalation. Eliminate even the pause between inhalation and exhalation.

In summary, the exercise goes as follows:

8 breaths lying on your back

16 breaths lying on your right side

32 breaths lying on your left side.

Very few people are able to finish this exercise before they drift into a restful sleep.

CHAPTER 5
The Mind and Stress

John Harvey, Ph.D.

The mind plays a paramount role in the problem of
stress. Ultimately, it is our appraisal of inner and outer
events that determines the nature and intensity of the stress
response. Once such an appraisal is made at conscious and
unconscious levels of the mind, the stress response follows.
The limbic system, the emotional center of the brain, is
activated, and then the autonomic nervous system, the
muscles, and the endocrine gland system move into action
and the concerted result is a full physiological stress response. It is this activity of the mind that can maintain this
response over time.

The importance of the mind in stress was quite clear to
Hans Selye, the founder of stress research, who in writing
about such stress-related diseases as hypertension, coronary
heart diseases, peptic ulcers, migraine headaches, and aches
and pain states emphatically: "These and many other diseases are not the direct results of any pathogen but of our
defective bodily or mental reactions to the stressors en-
countered in daily life."[1] Selye then provides a dramatic

This chapter is based on an article that appeared under the same title in
Dawn *magazine, Vol. 2, No. 2, 1982*

illustration of a definite, stress-producing reaction:

> "When you meet a helpless drunk who showers you with insults but is obviously quite unable to do you any harm, nothing will happen if you take a syntoxic attitude—go past and ignore him. However, if you respond catatoxically and fight, or even only prepare to fight, the consequence may be tragic. You will discharge adrenaline that increases blood pressure and pulse rate, while your whole system becomes alarmed and tense in anticipation of combat. If you happen to be a coronary candidate, the result may be a fatal heart accident. In this case who is the murderer? The drunk didn't even touch you. This is biological suicide. Death was caused by choosing the wrong reaction."[2]

Selye writes, further, that the secret of effective regulation of stress is based on a thoroughgoing analysis of our mental patterns. According to Selye, we need to cultivate the ability to experience inner peace and then to live and express a philosophy of purposeful altruism and social harmony.[3]

Other issues regarding the role of the mind in stress have been described by research psychologist George Mandler.[4] He notes that an important underlying dimension of our cognitive appraisal of events relates to the issue of mastery and control. When our appraisal enhances our sense of mastery and control, the resulting emotional tone is positive, and stress is minimized. For example, a white water canoe trip might be experienced as exhilarating because we have chosen to do it and have control over many aspects of the trip. Critical comments from a peer may be seen as positive if we think that the criticism will contribute to our mastery of the topic at hand. Yet, with a different appraisal, one of threat and loss of control, both the canoe trip and the critique could produce negative emotions, including anger, fear, sadness, frustration, and even terror. These emotions could in turn set off the stress response. The point is clear: it is our perspective on things, our mental appraisal of external events and external arousal, that determines our emotional tone and our levels of stress.

While contemporary researchers such as Selye and Mandler have pointed out the primacy of the mind in creating stress, ancient traditions of self-unfoldment such as yoga have always emphasized the understanding that the mind alone is the source of human suffering. Accordingly, within the tradition of yoga the control and regulation of mental activity is an essential step on the path of achieving optimal health and fostering self-development. Many methods and techniques have been developed to achieve mental balance and harmony. However, before we can utilize these valuable methods we must understand how mind is defined and the true nature of mental control.

In yoga mind is known as the inner instrument or *antah karana.* Mind is something unique. It stands between and at the same time connects our most essential being with what is external. It is in this way that mind is the finest instrument of our inner self, and yet through the activity of the thoughts and senses, we come to know and express ourself in the world of experience. The analogy is often given that the mind is like a lake. The bed of the lake is our essential self, the water is the mind stuff, and the waves, currents and turbulence in the water represent our thoughts, feelings, and memories.

Mind is also defined by the way it functions. In the science of yoga, four functions of mind are described. These are memory, sensory motor control, ego, and intellect. The memory function, known as *citta,* operates as a vast storehouse where mental impressions from previous experience are stored. The sensory motor function of the mind, known as *manas,* coordinates the activity of the sensory channels and directs motor behavior according to learned and habitual patterns. *Ahamkara* or the "I" sense is involved in determining and maintaining our unique sense of identity. *Buddhi* or intellect is known as the higher mind and involves the functions of will, logical thinking, decisiveness, and intuition. These four functional aspects of mind then work together to provide us with both conscious and unconscious mental experience.

Mind evolves from spirit and yet operates in the world of material experience. So mind is part of something higher; it is transcendent. Yet at the same time it is involved in sensory experience and in managing physiological function. This understanding allows the yogis to say that the whole of the body is in the mind, yet the whole of the mind is not in the body. Mind is like a subtle force that finds its expression in the complex workings of the brain and that presides over the symphonic functioning of the various physical systems. Consequently, when the mind is controlled, both brain and body are regulated.

But we must more carefully consider the nature of mental control. Control of the mind does not refer to some automatic process like switching a light on and off as if we can turn on and off harmful thought patterns. It is rather a process of directing the activity of the mind. Control in this sense means that we are aware of and then exercise choices in terms of mental activity. We direct the mind away from patterns that create suffering and stress toward patterns that lead us to health and self-unfoldment. There are many ways in which we expand our choices and learn to direct the mind, but for practical purposes it may be useful to consider three dimensions of mental functioning where we can learn an array of healthy patterns. These three dimensions are mental content, mental process, and mental structure.

Mental content refers to the habitual beliefs, attitudes, and self-talks that we utilize to evaluate inner and outer events. Mental process refers to such inner dynamics as attachments, fears, and identifications, around which content organizes. Mental structure addresses the actual condition or state of the mind. For example, is the mind focused or is it distracted? We will explore each of these dimensions in some detail, looking at dysfunctional and stress-producing patterns and then examining ways to reduce stress and promote health. Let us begin with the most accessible and malleable level of mind, that of mental content.

An example may serve to illustrate the effect of mental content. Imagine that two workers are performing their tasks at the same work bench. The foreman approaches and stands beside the table, not saying a word. Worker A is an anxious person and a perfectionist who can't stand criticism. Furthermore, he was brought up in a strict family and has a fear of authority figures. Recently he made several unfortunate errors on setting up a new job and wasted a considerable amount of time and money. On top of all this, his wife lost her job last week, and one of his children needs some expensive medical treatment. Worker B, on the other hand, is an easygoing fellow who seems to have a knack for negotiating and compromising. He is able to handle most situations with some humor. His early family life fostered self-respect and self-esteem. He is a close personal friend of the foreman and yesterday their families went on a picnic together and had a great time. Finally, Worker B has just accepted a job with another company that will give him more responsibility and a higher salary.

Both workers A and B are receiving the same sensory input: both view the foreman and wait for him to speak. Yet we can easily imagine that their emotional responses, subsequent physiological reactions, and resulting behaviors will be quite different. We might expect that worker A will feel a sense of dread; he will see a threat, and inwardly a stress response will result. His heart rate will increase, his hands will become cold, his mouth dry. In terms of behavior, he may become flustered and make errors at his work. Worker B, on the other hand, will most likely experience a positive emotional state. He may find a smile coming to his lips as he thinks of some of yesterday's jokes and good times. In terms of behavior, he is likely to be relaxed and friendly.

Thus, there are two radically different interpretations of the same stimulus event. These differing perceptions seem to be the result of many factors, including early childhood experiences, personality traits, and the entire context of the situation. Perhaps we can capture this relationship by the use of diagrams. For the sake of convenience, let us assume that all sensory impressions are processed through an interpretive filter before we have a response.

Figure 1 illustrates this filter. It can be seen that we interpret all stimulus input, including both outer and inner events, and this filtering is what causes our responses. Typically, an emotional response involves three components: our feelings, a physiological reaction (flight or fight or possum response), and a behavioral response. Clearly this complex emotional response is determined by how we filter events. Ultimately, then, our filter determines whether or not we experience mental and physiological imbalance. Since this filtering or interpreting capacity of the mind is so important, let us consider it in somewhat greater detail. Figure 1 shows some of the components of the filter. As we can see, some of them are more conscious and available to us than are others. The most available level is what we might call self-talks. This is the realm of conscious interpretation.

We continually talk to ourselves throughout the day. If we step back and listen for a few seconds, we can notice a kind of internal, running commentary. We talk to ourselves as we're driving: "Look at that fool, speeding like

Figure 1

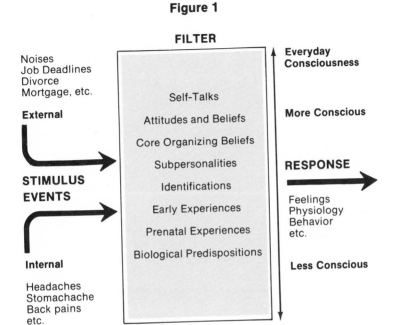

that; I hope he doesn't try to cut me off." We talk to ourselves when we wash the dishes: "I can't wait to finish; I think I'll have a nice cup of tea when I'm done." We talk to ourselves about our memories and sensations and about events in the world around us. By means of these self-talks, we evaluate our sense impressions.

Therefore, the content of this inner talk influences the way we respond and the level of stress we experience. One researcher in the area of stress management, Hermann Witte, has discovered that people who experience stress differ from those who don't have stress primarily on the basis of their self-talks.[5] Witte has distinguished two broad categories of people on this basis. "Thin-skinned" people tend to have habitual self-talks that lead them to overreact to inner and outer events. These people "stress" themselves into illness. The second category is "thick-skinned" people, whose self-talks lead to a much more balanced and ultimately more happy and productive life. The goal in stress management is to rid ourselves of these thin-skinned self-talks. Before we can do this, however, there are several basic assumptions that we need to examine. The first of these assumptions addresses the issue of causation in emotions. There are basically two models of causation: "It upsets me," and "I upset myself." The "It upsets me" model maintains that a stimulus event necessarily leads us to experience a certain emotion. In other words, if someone rejects us, we must feel sad and worthless; if we are fired from our job, we must feel bad—the situation or the event determines our emotions. People who accept this model characteristically blame other people and external factors for their upsets. Their coping strategies are all outwardly directed: they try to cope either by escaping the situation or by attacking the person or situation that they view as being the cause of their upset.

The view that "It upsets me" tends to overlook the role of our cognitive filter. When we accept the notion of "I upset myself," we then recognize the controlling role of our filtering, interpreting mind. As we accept this view, we can take responsibility for our emotions, and we can begin to look within for change. Many people find it hard to accept the notion that they are responsible for their emotions. Yet if we carefully examine two lines of evidence we will recognize that we are indeed responsible for upsetting ourselves.

The first line of evidence is that the same stimulus event can cause different responses in different people. In a thousand different people, the sight of a snake can create a thousand different responses, on a continuum from absolute terror to curiosity to pleasure. The snake doesn't *create* those different responses; it is the human interpretation, appraisal, and self-talks that create the response. The same is true for the workers A and B we mentioned earlier because the foreman is simply there. It is each worker's own internal processing and self-talks that determine the emotional response and ultimately the stress level that he experiences.

The second point is that as we look at our life experiences, we can notice that our reactions to any one event change over time. Perhaps we used to become angry and defensive when someone criticized us, and now it doesn't bother us, because we have changed our filter and self-talks for this stimulus event. We simply don't upset ourselves about criticism any more. Conversely, there may be things that never bothered us before but that now irritate or even anger us greatly. Again, the event is the same but our self-talks have changed.

Most people need a good deal of time and experience before they fully accept the idea that they upset themselves. But this concept is the starting point for managing stress (imbalance) in the mind. We should also consider this "response-ability" in a positive light: it means that we have a choice and that we are "able to respond" differently in the future.

✳ Once we have grasped the notion of "I upset myself," there are several other assumptions we can use to help promote change. The first of these is that the vast majority of our self-talks are learned. We learn them in our family life, from our friends, and from society. If indeed the self-talks that create stress are learned, then we can learn new ones that will allow us to respond in a more balanced manner.

Initially, we may feel quite different when we use new self-talks and respond with relative calmness to a situation that previously caused anger and frustration. We may feel phony and unlike the self we know, but this is simply a case of the old pattern having created a groove in our mind. We know the old way of responding and are comfortable with it. When we choose new self-talks and experience a healthier emotional response it may seem unfamiliar, but if we persist it will come to feel quite natural to use our new self-talks to maintain a more positive and balanced outlook on events.

It is also important to recognize the difference between primary coping and secondary coping. Primary coping involves our immediate reaction to a stressor. If this stressor is a significant life event (for example, signing a mortgage, the death of a family member, or losing or starting a job), we will expect to see significant emotional activation. The difficulty comes with secondary coping. Do we get over the shock and rebalance our emotions and behavior, or do we continue to experience upset over a long period of time? In fact, as time goes on, does our thin-skinned thinking about the event actually lead us to more emotional upset and greater stress?

Let us illustrate this point with an example. Suppose someone is unexpectedly fired from his job. His first reaction is one of shock and disbelief. Then he may feel some anger and anxiety, but this lasts only a day or two. By the third day the person has reconciled himself to the reality of being fired, has stopped condemning himself, and has begun to map out a strategy for finding a new and perhaps more satisfying job. This would be an example of typical primary coping (emotional upset) followed by useful secondary coping (managing to regain balance in the realms of feelings, physiology, and behavior).

The person with poor secondary coping would have a basically different response following the initial upset. He might withdraw and brood on his failure and, as a result, upset both his physiology and his family life. He might continue to blame and berate himself for his incompetence and at the same time seethe with anger about the lack of understanding that his boss showed. As a consequence, he might begin to suffer from stomach problems or headaches that would then make it even more difficult to undertake any new activities. The person with poor secondary coping skills not only fails to rebalance but actually creates additional problems for himself. A significant difference between those who have good secondary coping skills and those who don't lies in their self-talks, their differing ways of interpreting events over time.

It might be useful at this point to recast our various assumptions about the nature of self-talks into four positive statements. These are:

1. Only I can upset myself, which I do with my self-talks.

2. My self talks are learned and I can learn new ones.

3. Although it may be difficult to change old patterns, with effort and persistence I can change.

4. Ultimately I can regulate the nature, intensity and duration of my emotional responses.

With these assumptions as a foundation we are ready to begin addressing specific patterns of self-talks and replacing any dysfunctional and stress-producing thoughts with functional and health-enhancing thoughts.

Categories of Self-Talks

Stress-producing self-talks may be placed in six distinct categories.[6] We will describe and discuss each of these categories in detail. The first category may be defined as demandingness, and involves rigid, unrealistic demands that we make of others, of ourselves, and of life in general. In our inner language we frequently couch these demands in terms such as *should, must,* and *have to.* When we phrase our expectations in these terms, we have created rigid demands, and when our demands are not met, we experience upset. It is this upset and our subsequent elaboration of it that is the cause of stress. It will therefore be of considerable value to analyze our mental habit of demandingness.

There are three broad classes of demands. The first

involves the demands that we make upon others. Typically we have certain expectations of our family members, our co-workers, our neighbors, the people who sell us things, our leaders, and so on. We have expectations of almost everyone we interact with. When these expectations are framed in the language of rigid demands, we tell ourselves that, for example, our spouse *should* understand us, that our children *must* obey us, that our colleagues *have to* respect us, that our boss *should* treat us fairly, that sales-people *must* be polite. When these demands are not met, we feel angry, hurt, frustrated, and sad.

Frequently, we support our demands with what seem to be very sound reasons. We note that we wouldn't behave in an inconsiderate manner and believe that, therefore, others shouldn't. Perhaps we see others' behavior as contrary to the Ten Commandments and other ethical codes, and feel that we are justified in condemning their behavior and expecting them to change. This reasoning, although plausible at first glance, is unrealistic: people ultimately behave according to their own impulses. People behave the way they want to and not the way we want them to.

This leads us to a crucial point. A rigid expectation is really nothing more than a rationalized desire. Simply put, we would prefer others to behave in a certain way, and we then encode this, with the help of some pompous reasoning, into the categorical imperative that they should or must behave in a certain way. To reprogram our thinking, we must go back to our original desire. It will help us to recognize that we simply want or prefer something. With this in mind we can approach others in a more flexible manner, for we all realize that we simply don't get everything we want, especially from others.

From the perspective of yoga psychology, desires and the ensuing attachments are indeed at the root of emotional imbalance. *Shoulds, musts,* and *have-tos* are the language of emotional attachment to and dependence upon people and external objects. As we temper our inner language, we weaken the attachment and also become more independent of the desire. When we truly believe that we would only prefer or like something, we become more free and nonattached. We no longer need to have this desire satisfied to feel whole and complete. Consequently, we are much more likely to experience contentment and emotional balance.

It is also useful to consider our own motives and needs. In any cluster of dysfunctional self-talks, there is always some underlying emotional hook. In the case of expectations toward others, we frequently find the need for acceptance and recognition. To some degree, our sense of self is contingent upon this acceptance or recognition. We have an externally conditioned sense of self, and consequently our self-concept is based on external factors such as recognition, praise, and acceptance from others. This tends to make us addicted to these external factors; we feel that we must have this acceptance, control, and recognition. And when it doesn't come as we expect, we experience emotional upset.

Breaking these emotional addictions and making our self-talks more thick-skinned involves several steps. To begin, we can revise our self-talks into the language of preferences and wants. We can begin to tell ourselves that while we might like acceptance and we might prefer to have recognition or control, that we don't have to have these things to survive. Obviously, it becomes easier to adopt such constructive and flexible self-talks when we are able to foster an abiding sense of self-worth.

A second group of rigid demands concerns the expectations we place on ourselves. These self-expectations, which are quite common, revolve around acceptance, control, performance, and competence. Examples are "I must succeed," "I must do things correctly," or "I should never make mistakes." These are thin-skinned self-talks that lead us to stress. Typically, such rigid self-demands lead us to critically monitor our behavior in a manner that may actually interfere with performance. Then, as our performance falters, we create anger and disgust within ourselves. Guilt sets in, and in extreme instances we become paralyzed with helplessness (the possum response) and the conviction that we can't do anything.

Many of the self-expectations that we carry around are picked up from family and society. Over the course of time we come to believe that we should and must behave in a certain way. When we begin to examine our own rigid self-expectations, a first question is to determine if we really want to be that way. Often we find that we don't. For example, we may have been telling ourselves that we should make a lot of money and gain status and recognition. Yet, when we examine these issues we find that, in fact, these are not our most important goals. Getting rid of such automatic expectations alleviates much inner conflict. It helps us to recast our self-expectations into the form of softer, more realistic wants and preferences. When we see them in this light, two things tend to happen. First, we become more accepting when we don't fulfill our own expectations. A therapist, for example, might acknowledge, "I would like to help each client, but in fact I may not help every client as much as I'd like to." Second, when we clearly recognize that we do want something and become more conscious of this want, it can become an ideal. An ideal that is free of fantasy and sheer imagination, has the capacity to make our personality healthy. We may have feelings of hope, enthusiasm, and energy in regard to an ideal. These are strengthening, healing emotions that lead us toward a more dynamic emotional state.

The third type of rigid demand involves expectations about life in general. We have beliefs about the way things should be for us in the world. Examples of these self-talks are: "Life should go smoothly; I shouldn't have to deal with excessive problems and difficulties."

And then, unfortunately, when our car breaks down or the basement is flooded, we become upset because we believe and then demand that such things shouldn't happen. The fact is that such things can and do happen. There is, in fact, no guarantee that any of us should be spared life's problems, be they as minor as a leaking faucet or as weighty as the loss of a loved one. All human beings experience tragedies and difficulties in life. Opening up and accepting the possibility that these things can happen to us allows us to accept hard times when they come and to do our conscious best to avoid difficulties. In a surprising and paradoxical manner, opening up to the problematic side of life allows us to glean whatever of value might come from hard times and to more totally embrace that which is positive in life.

Denial is a second major category of stress-producing self-talks. Denial typically follows demandingness and compounds its effect by increasing negative emotions. There are actually two aspects to denial. The first is denying that something happened whereas the second is denying insight into the event. In the first case we generate such self-talks as, "I can't believe this is happening" or, "I just can't believe that he did that." Repeating such self-talks simply heightens our upset. We can deal with this type of denial by doing a reality check. We must ask ourselves, did the event happen or not? If indeed it did, if we can verify that it occurred, then we can accept it.

Overcoming the tendency to deny insight is slightly more complex. This type of denial is characterized by such self-talks as, "I can't understand why she did that" or, "I can't believe I did that." As we repeat such statements to ourselves we feel all the more perplexed, anxious, and upset. We can begin to gain insight by reminding ourselves that the causes behind events are often not readily apparent. It may require some time and persistent effort on our part to unravel the reasons for our behavior or the behavior of someone else. And if we really want to understand why something happened we can study the event, contemplate our motivation, and gather information from others. In the meantime we can help ourselves by accepting the fact that both we and others often behave in an impulsive or even automatic manner. Acknowledging this impulsiveness and automaticity can dramatically reduce excessive negative emotions.

Perhaps a brief exercise can help us see how acceptance and insight can reduce our negative emotions. Consider someone who has made you quite angry during the last week. Think about what he or she did and re-examine your response—feelings, physical reactions, and behavior. Now, imagine that this person went to a prestigious hospital for a week and underwent a through medical evaluation. The results of this checkup indicate that the person has a small benign brain tumor. This is not a dangerous tumor and doesn't require any surgery, but because of its location and size it has a predictable effect on behavior. In fact, this tumor has caused and will cause the person to do exactly the kind of thing that prompted your anger. Given this knowledge, what happens to the negative emotions? Typically they are dramatically reduced because our self-talks change instantly. We say to ourselves, "He has a brain tumor and can't help himself." We may even feel some compassion, but we definitely have a different understanding of why he acted the way he did. We no longer blame this person. Our anger decreases—we don't take his behavior personally.

Fortunately, such physical tumors are rare, but what we might call psychological brain tumors are quite common. Many people respond in counter-productive, selfish, or unfortunate ways. But if we have the ability to recognize that it is just their brain tumor acting up, we can maintain our emotional balance. From a point of balance, we can more effectively accept what is and work on changing what we don't like. It may be useful to add that as we come to recognize the brain tumors of others, we can also acknowledge our own brain tumors, accept our own impulsive behavior without excessive self-condemnation, and respond differently in the future.

The third major category of disturbing self-talks is called overreacting and it involves the way we evaluate things when our expectations are not met. Typically, in these situations we overreact. We tend to "horribilize" things; when something contrary to our expectations occurs, we tell ourselves, "It's horrible, I can't stand it." The event might be something relatively minor, such as a traffic jam, waiting in line, or criticism from a friend. Nevertheless, if we continually flash the message in the cerebral cortex, "It's horrible, I can't stand it!" our autonomic nervous system and endocrine glands begin to respond as though the event is a true emergency. This happens because our inner physiology does not have direct sensory input; it relies on the decision-making of our conscious mind. Therefore, whenever we overreact we also produce an excessive response from our inner physiology, with a resultant state of imbalance and stress.

Consider the following analogy. Imagine the body as a great fortress; on the top of the fortress is a watchtower and control room, which represent the senses and the brain. Deep within the fort is an engine room, where all the heating, air-conditioning, and electrical generation equipment is housed. These systems are analogous to the autonomic nervous system and the endocrine system. The functioning of these important systems depends upon the information received and the decisions made in the control room. The engine room itself has no direct contact with the outside world, and depends upon the watchtower and control room in order to activate properly and to know when maintenance can be carried out.

Let us imagine a scenario where the person on duty in the watchtower continuously activates an emergency response for rather minor problems. If there is a slight draft the heating system is brought up to a maximum level, and if the sun shines too warmly through one window the air-conditioning is turned up to a maximum value. And anytime the least little threat is seen, a general alarm is sounded. The resources of the fortress are being squandered by the tendency to overreact in the watchtower and control room.

An analogous situation occurs when we continually overreact to events in our daily life. Our nervous and endocrine systems depend on the decisions and cognitive evaluations made in the brain. These, in turn, are based on the words we use to evaluate outer and inner events. Words are highly efficient and effective mobilizers of our autonomic nervous system and our endocrine system.

Over time, through our life experiences and the modeling of family and friends, words come to take on emotional meanings. We develop conditioned emotional responses. There are whole groups of words that, when used in the watchtower of our mind, act to set off, maintain, and heighten negative emotions. These involve such words as "awful," "terrible," and "miserable," and include such patterns as, "I can't stand it," "It drains me," "It tears me up," "It kills me," and "It breaks my heart." These words and statements have a powerful emotional effect. When we continually use them to respond to the ups and downs of life, we activate our body and nervous system and eventually create health problems. On the other hand, by choosing different self-talks we have an opportunity to regulate our emotional response to life events and to protect our health.

There are a couple of key points that can support our move to choosing better words. The first is that nothing is inherently horrible or terrible. Something simply exists; it is merely there. We assign a value to it. If we look at our own experience we can see that the way we evaluate events can change. For example, time has a great "dehorribilizing" effect. Something that was terribly upsetting ten years ago can often be viewed with greater equanimity now. This is because we have more distance and a wider perspective on the issue. We no longer label it as horrible. We see it with greater dispassion, and feel less emotional addiction. We can use the perspective of time to cope better with upsetting life events by employing what is known as the "six-by-six" test. We can ask ourselves, while in the throes of overreacting to some event, how we might feel about it six years from now. If we believe that we will feel less upset, then we can ask ourselves how we will feel in six months. Again, we may realize that in six months the event won't bother us much at all. And then we can continue to move the time frame closer to the present asking the same question for six weeks, six days, six hours, and even six minutes. Invariably the six-by-six procedure helps us reduce negative emotions and stress. We may find ourselves employing such coping self-talks as, "I may not like what has happened but I certainly can deal with it and know I'll get over it."

Another way to dehorribilize is to utilize *reframing*— that is, to attempt to assign a different meaning to events. For example, if we reflect on our own past we can often find an event such as a job loss or the ending of a relationship that seemed truly horrible when we experienced it. As we look back now on the event, we realize that it was a valuable turning point. In the case of losing a job, this change might have provided the opportunity to assess our interests and to move into a much more challenging and satisfying job. Or we might now realize that by leaving a relationship, we had the opportunity to develop other relationships that have been far more rewarding.

This reframing of a seemingly negative event deals

with what might be called "the silver lining effect." The saying is that "every dark cloud has a silver lining." This principle is recognized in the Chinese language, where the character representing "crisis" is a composite of two characters, one meaning "danger" and the other meaning "opportunity." Reframing means to grasp the opportunity. It means attuning ourselves to the positive potential in any situation. It means looking for the opportunities in learning and growth in any crisis.

As we learn to use the techniques of time distancing and reframing, we will find ourselves reacting in a more balanced manner. We will begin to evaluate situations using self-talks that sound like this:

"Perhaps it's unfortunate and unpleasant, but surely not horrible."

"Even though I may be somewhat uncomfortable about this event, I can be open to the potential for learning, positive change, and personal growth that this event may bring with it."

"Dehorribilizing" may be quite challenging in the face of major life events, such as divorce, terminal illness, the death of a loved one, or a tragic accident. In this regard, a story about the Buddha is relevant. A women distraught about the death of her young son went to the Buddha and asked him to bring her son back to life. He agreed to do this if the woman could procure some mustard seeds from a house that had never been visited by death. She went busily from house to house and, after some time, discovered that her search was in vain. She then returned to the Buddha ready to accept the passing of her son, and to move ahead with her life. Certainly no one can be free from sad life events. What we can do is to choose those self-talks that prevent us from getting excessively upset about these events and work to accept them as gracefully as possible.

A fourth major category of disturbing and stress-producing self-talks is "always" and "never" thinking. Self-talks in this category concern our perspective on the future. We often project our emotional upset into the future and then reinforce this projection with the use of "always" and "never" self-talks. Because some negative event occurs now, we tell ourselves it will always happen in the future. Because we have been rejected, made an error at work, or feel sad, we tell ourselves that in the future we will always be rejected, make work errors, or feel sad. When we feel alone and dissatisfied with ourselves, when we fail to achieve our goals, we tell ourselves that we will never feel fulfilled and that we will never achieve our goals. Such self-talks give our nervous system a powerful yet contradictory message. On the one hand, we activate the nervous system because things aren't the way we demand they should be, but on the other hand, we shut down because we are convinced that there is nothing we can do. This is comparable to trying to drive away from danger by pushing the accelerator and brakes of a car simultaneously. It does little good, and may damage the car as well.

There are a number of methods for ridding ourselves of the unfortunate habit of always-and-never thinking. The first approach is to understand the nature of emotions: unless reinforced by the wrong self-talks, feelings tend to come and go rather quickly. In Eastern psychology, the changeable nature of emotions is well understood. Emotions are often compared to a river. If we stand calmly on the bank, we will notice that the river constantly changes. Even the mightiest of floods is followed by a return to a more moderate water level in time. It is the nature of emotions to change. If we can train ourselves to observe our feelings rather than being obsessed with them, we can re-establish emotional balance sooner. If we can stand back and let the feelings pass rather than identifying with them we can cultivate a healthy and realistic set of self-talks about our feelings. We can come to tell ourselves that "This, too, shall pass." Then when confronted with a difficult situation or bad times, we can avoid overreacting and projecting our plight into the interminable future, and instead regain our emotional balance.

Another method for overcoming always-and-never thinking is to regain a personal sense of control in those areas where we can exercise some control. We can carefully survey our situation and identify actions that we might take to begin to improve things. The key is to focus on small manageable steps that can begin the process of improvement. It is astounding how much better we feel when we are taking some action to help ourselves. And, of course, as soon as we begin to do something we are defeating the logic of always-and-never thinking. We can also increase our psychological hardiness by cultivating a personal philosophy that acknowledges that it is our essential birthright to have hope. We can strengthen this sense of hope by looking at the lives of great people and seeing how they persisted even in the face of significant obstacles. And we can find examples of people confronted with tragedy who have continued to find meaning, satisfaction, and happiness in life. We can also look back at our own lives, recalling the times we have overcome obstacles and dealt with tragedies, and then, regain our strength to do the same in the present and future. The important role of hope in overcoming stress is discussed in greater detail in Chapter 11 of this book entitled "Stress, Helplessness, and Hope."

The fifth major category of stress-producing self-talks is all-or-nothing thinking. Here, we see some fault in ourselves or others and generalize beyond it to create a global evaluation. The reasoning goes something like this: "Because I made a mistake on this job I am a totally incompetent person." We also apply the same thinking to others. Because they don't live up to our demands they are rotten, ill-tempered, and inconsiderate people. This type of all-or-nothing thinking is based on the "behavior equals the person" fallacy: <u>one negative behavior makes our perception of the person negative.</u> This type of thinking increases and maintains anger, frustration, disgust, and hopelessness. It dramatically impairs self-esteem. It also inhibits our ability to solve problems, look for alternative solutions, and be aware of the positive aspects of ourselves and of others.

Logic can help us overcome the tendency to engage in all-or-nothing thinking; it does not follow that because others do something we don't like, they are worthless, despicable, or rotten. Such thinking is overgeneralizing and is illogical. We are using one piece of evidence to create a whole picture. Even if there is one aspect to a situation that we don't like there are likely to be many more that are positive and likeable.

We need to maintain a balanced perspective. No matter how significant the error we or someone else makes, we can't ignore a person's—or our own—basic value as a human being. This broader perspective allows us to feel less anger towards them. In the throes of cutting ourselves to shreds over some mistake, perhaps we can regain a sense of hope and a feeling of energy. By keeping a balanced perspective and avoiding overgeneralizing we are able to deal more effectively with the incident or problem at hand. Free from the grasp of excessive emotionality, we can observe our own problem behavior as interesting, study its causes and effects, and consider ways to do things differently in the future. In a similar vein, if we can avoid global condemnations of others, we can focus instead on the specific behaviors and begin to ask for and negotiate change.

Ultimately, our self-esteem, self-confidence, and creative will are crucial factors necessary in the journey of life. Equally important is our sense of community with others. Both self-regard and community with others are weakened by unreasonable all-or-nothing thinking. Overcoming this type of fallacious all-or-nothing thinking is crucial in reducing stress, protecting our health, and developing our potential. Changes in our self-talks will certainly allow us to overcome the habit of all-or-nothing thinking and to utilize our emotional energy in much more constructive ways.

The sixth major category of stress-producing self-talks concerns our thoughts and beliefs about the opinions of others. "Mind-reading" is a good label for this group of self-talks because we believe we know exactly what others are thinking about us. Actually there are two types of mind reading. The first involves assumptions regarding what others are perceiving and the second involves beliefs about how others are evaluating us. In the first case, we imagine that others are noticing every aspect of our current mental, emotional, and physical state. If, for example, we are feeling anxious, we "know" that others are aware of our nervousness, tension, pounding heart, and sweaty palms. And if we are feeling guilty, we know that others can read this feeling.

The second type of mind-reading then follows from this quite naturally. We believe we know how others are evaluating us. If they perceive our anxiety, then they are thinking that we are a nervous and weak person. If they recognize our guilt, then they are thinking that we are weak, guilt-ridden, and incompetent. Sometimes this second type of mind-reading occurs when we believe that others are making negative evaluations of us based on our behavior. For example, if we do something careless or impulsive, then we believe that others evaluate us as a careless, incompetent, and generally worthless person. We make ourselves even more upset when we believe that these negative evaluations by others are permanent and unchanging.

Mind-reading adds to our stress in a number of ways. First of all, it leads us to generate a number of the previously discussed self-talks. For example, if we believe that others can see our anxiety and evaluate us as incompetent, we may engage in horribilizing. And we may engage in always-never thinking to the effect that others will always see us as ineffective and that we will never be accepted. Mind-reading also promotes a kind of negative self-watching where we are constantly concerned about our performance. We fear the slightest error, as it may worsen others' opinions of us. Accordingly, we become much more self-conscious and tense when we are around others and more likely to make mistakes. And as we are preoccupied with others' negative evaluations we actually cut ourselves off from perceiving and accepting the positive and supportive evaluations that others in fact may be making. Consequently, mind-reading contributes to our inner turmoil and isolates us from others. This type of thinking definitely adds to our stress and it can be quite helpful to break out of this harmful pattern.

There are several ways to confront and change mind-reading. The first is to challenge the assumption that others are really able to perceive our inner states. The fact is, our inner signals of distress are much louder and more apparent to us than to others. We can hear and feel the pounding of our heart, the tremor in our voice, and the shakiness of our limbs. But these same signals are barely perceptible to others. As a frequent public speaker, there have been occasions when I felt nervous while speaking and was convinced that this was readily apparent to all in attendance. To say the least, I was surprised when people in the audience would comment after my talk that they had noticed how calm I was. It was clear to me that they simply were not aware of my inner experience of tension. Their perceptions were, most likely, influenced by their own mindset and expectations. And if they did notice some signs of tension, it is quite likely that they didn't dwell on them. Ultimately, their attention was dominated by their own concerns, issues, and physical experiences.

A second assumption to challenge is the belief that others are automatically thinking something negative about us. The fact of the matter is that their evaluations can run the gamut from positive to neutral to negative. It is reasonable to assume that others' evaluations are divided equally across these three categories. This means that probably at least one third of the time people are viewing us in a positive manner. They may be sympathizing with us in distress or applauding our successes. To believe that others are seeing us only in a negative manner is a projection of our own doubts and insecurities. On the basis of chance, we could assume that another third of the time people see us in a neutral light. One of the main reasons for this is that they are preoccupied with their own interests and doubts.

Finally, there may be instances where others do evaluate us negatively. Then it is important for us to cultivate several healthy attitudes, including the belief that what others think is not truly important. A study of the lives of great and effective people will show that they always had critics and detractors. Of course, it is pleasant to have people like us and to be regarded positively, but it is not life-threatening if we are not. We also need to recall that people's opinions change in the most surprising manner. Time and circumstance can bring the bitterest of enemies into close friendships. And in a more immediate sense, be assured that if you win two million dollars in the lottery today, by tomorrow many critics will suddenly become your friend.

It is simply not healthy or logical to become too worried about the evaluations of others. At times we can gain valuable feedback and input by listening to others. If we have doubts or questions about what others are thinking, we can ask them—we may be surprised to discover how often these evaluations are supportive and positive.

Even if someone does have a negative opinion of us, we can endure it. In fact, we may be able to reframe it and learn something from the experience. There is a saying that one learns much more from his enemies than from his friends. In any event, it is helpful to discard mind-reading self-talks that only contribute to stress and to develop instead healthy and realistic beliefs about the opinions of others.

We have now identified and discussed six major categories of self-talks that initiate, maintain, and intensify the negative emotions of stress. These six are: demandingness, denial, overreacting, always-never thinking, all-or-nothing thinking, and mind-reading. In each case we have looked at how these self-talks arise, and at the reasoning that supports them. Most importantly, for each category we have examined ways to dispute these stress producing self-talks and to develop more flexible, healthy, and coping self-talks.

The next step is to become adept at recognizing and revising our self-talks during the often hectic and pressured flow of daily life. This requires practice. A systematic procedure that can be employed to gain experience and skill in revising disturbing self-talks is given below. This procedure will make it much easier to subsequently recognize and change stress producing self-talks throughout the day and in any situation.

Changing Self-Talks

To revise our self-talks we might remind ourselves of the relationship between events, thoughts, and emotions. To recapitulate, something happens either inside of us or in our environment, and the way that we perceive, think about, and evaluate it determines our emotional reaction.  If our thinking and evaluating are dysfunctional, we wind up with an excessive emotional response and the end result is stress. An example of a dysfunctional response to an event is shown in the top half of Table 1 on pp. 114-15. The self-talks are placed in six columns according to the six major categories described above. The emotional response is divided into the components of feelings, physiological changes, and behaviors. The feelings are rated on a scale of 1-10 with 10 indicating the highest possible intensity.

In the bottom half of the table the self-talks are revised according to the perspectives described in the previous section of this chapter. Thus, the emotional response is considerably moderated, the degree of stress is reduced, and the behavioral response is more likely to solve problems rather than to accentuate them.

Several points should be noted concerning Table 1. First of all, this table represents a snapshot of emotional life, in which a moment is frozen in time so that we can study and analyze it. In actuality, emotional processing is fluid and dynamic. Feelings, physiology, and behavior, as well as the ever-changing environment, all act as stimuli for additional evaluation and continual emotional response. Emotions function more as ongoing patterns than as isolated events. Nevertheless, it can be useful to take such a snapshot, analyze it, and use it to revise our emotional response.

A second point is that the table highlights the individuality of our emotional patterns. Each person viewing the table may notice that certain of the self-talks are quite familiar and recognizable to him or her while others are not. Accordingly, it may be useful to focus on our own individual response pattern and our particular sensitive areas as we move ahead in the process of emotional self regulation.

This table can also be used as a worksheet to examine a given emotional response and then change it. You, the reader, will benefit in at least three ways if you perform this exercise. First, it will help you to cope more effectively with a specific event. Second, it illustrates the experience of witnessing, that is, observing your thought patterns and choosing more helpful ones. Third, when you practice this written exercise several times you will become more proficient in monitoring and changing your self-talks on an ongoing basis in the future. You will be able to note excessive negative reactions, identify the stress producing self-talks, and then change them in the flux and flow of daily life.

To begin, take a sheet of paper, divide it into eight columns, and then draw a line horizontally across the middle. Starting with the top left hand column, list an event that has recently created emotional upset for you. This event may be something that happened to you, such as a serious argument, a mistake at work, or someone failing to fulfill a promise. You may also be concerned by some internal event, such as a headache, stomach problems, or feelings of nervousness. The more recent the event and the stronger your feelings about it, the better target it is for successful revision. Try to get yourself into a witnessing mode where you can to some extent observe your inner thinking and feeling responses. If you are feeling very emotional about the event you may want to slow down your breathing and consciously relax the muscles. It is important to reduce the internal noise and distraction of a strong emotional response so that you can engage in some constructive self-study. The breathing and relaxation techniques discussed elsewhere in this book can be very useful in this regard.

Now, once you have described the event and calmed yourself to the point where you can observe what is happening inside yourself, describe your emotional response in the upper right hand column. First, list your feelings. If you are not sure what your feelings are, close your eyes and allow yourself to sense your spontaneous response to the event. Do you want to fight someone or do you want to run away? Do you feel sickened or do you want to cry? Such urges relate to the feelings of anger, fear, disgust, and sadness. Don't be surprised if there are a number of feelings. Most emotional responses are, in fact, a blend of feelings. In some cases there are layers of feelings. You may notice anger and then beneath that, hurt, and finally, sadness. Whatever feelings you have, they

Table 1

Event (Original)	Demands	Denial	Overreaction
Fired suddenly from job late one Friday afternoon.	The boss shouldn't have fired me. He should have been more understanding. He should know I have been trying to do my best. I should have handled the job. I shouldn't have made any mistakes. Things like this just shouldn't happen.	I can't believe this happened. I can't understand why he fired me. How could I let something like this happen to me?	This is terrible. I can't handle it. It's awful. This is ruining me. It's killing me. This is a catastrophe.
Event (Revised)	**Demands**	**Denial**	**Overreaction**
Fired suddenly from job late on Friday afternoon.	I would prefer not to be fired. I'd like it if the boss was more under-standing. I'd like to handle the job better. It would be nice if things like this didn't happen.	Did it happen? Yes, so I must accept that it has indeed happened. The boss must have had some reason for firing me. Perhaps I need to improve and maybe I can understand that.	This is unfortunate and inconvenient but I'm still alive and I can stand it even if I don't like it. Maybe there is even an opportunity for positive outcomes from the event. Perhaps I can learn something. If possible I will find a better job.

Always/Never	All/Nothing	Mind Reading	Emotional Response
I'll never get another job. I'll never be able to hold a job. I'll always be a failure. I'll always feel this depressed and angry. I always make mistakes. I can never handle difficult situations.	I'm a real loser. I'm a total failure. I'm good for nothing. My career is totally destroyed. The boss is an absolute jerk.	People can see how bad I feel. My neighbors think I'm a failure and they will put me down. All the people at work are putting me down.	*Feelings* Anger 8 Disgust 8 Frustration 8 Sadness 9 Hopelessness 9 *Physiology* Heart racing, diarrhea, mind racing, breath short, stomach in knots, neck hurts. *Behavior* Yell at family, avoid friends, drink too much, watch too much TV.
Always/Never	**All/Nothing**	**Mind Reading**	**Emotional Response**
What will this mean in 6 years? This too shall pass. Even my negative feelings will unwind. Just because I may have done something wrong on this job doesn't prove I always do things wrong. Let me think about what I can do to improve things from this point on.	I'm a fallible human being. I may make mistakes but this is just one thing and there are many things I do well. Essentially, I'm OK. While this may be a setback it doesn't mean my career is over. In fact, things might get better.	I don't know for sure what others are thinking. If I want to know, I'll ask. Actually they may be sympathetic or at worst, concerned with their own affairs. In any event, it doesn't matter, because others' opinions can change rapidly.	*Feelings* Anger 2 Disgust 2 Frustration 1 Sadness 3 Hopelessness 1 *Physiology* Slight headache, some fatigue, unsettled stomach. *Behavior* Initiate systematic job search. Start exercise program. Catch up on household projects. Evaluate work values and priorities.

are yours and they provide valuable information in the process of self-study. Once you have established and identified your feelings, rate them according to intensity, applying the 1-10 scale. As a general guideline, you can consider the possibility that a rating of six or above may represent the type of emotional response that creates stress. If you rate your feelings at an intensity of four or five it seems to indicate you are coping to some degree. If the intensity level is at three or below you are coping fairly well and you probably don't need to revise your self-talks.

Next, study your physiological response. What is going on with your muscles? Do you notice patterns of tightening anywhere in your body? Consider the reaction of the autonomic nervous system. Do you feel your heart beating more rapidly or is your stomach tied in knots? List all of the physical reactions of your emotional response. Finally, examine your behavioral response. What did you do in response to the event? Did you yell at someone or freeze up?

Once you have noted your behavior, then you have considered all three components of your emotional response—feelings, physiology, and behavior. Now, you are ready to work with the six remaining columns in between the event and the response. You can begin to discover what types of thoughts and beliefs led from the event to your response.

The remaining six columns may be labelled D1, D2, 0, AN1, AN2, and MR. These stand for the six major categories of stress producing self-talks discussed in the previous section. These are demands, denial, overreaction, always-never thinking, all-or-nothing thinking, and mind, reading. Go through each category, identifying the self-talks that create and maintain your emotional response. In the first column, note the rigid and inflexible demands that you are making of yourself, of others, and of life in general. Be aware of your thinking and see what kind of "shoulds" are setting off your response. In column two, examine the issue of denial. Are you accepting what has occurred? Can you begin to understand some of the possible causes for the event? Then, in the third column, under "O" examine your reaction to the event. Are you telling yourself that the event is interesting or are you engaging in overreacting and horribilizing about it?

As you consider the AN1 column, listen to the always-never thinking that may be going on inside your head. Are you projecting that this horrible state will always exist? Do you believe that either you, another person, or the situation itself can never change? Move on to the AN2 column and become aware of any all-or-nothing thinking. Are you describing either yourself or others as without value, totally unworthy of love, respect, or affection? Finally, in the last column, look for your patterns of mind reading. Write down any attributions you are making regarding the perceptions of others or any negative evaluations that you believe others are formulating about you.

When you have filled in all the columns you will have a good idea about the kinds of beliefs and self-talks that have created your stress-producing emotional response. Now you can begin to revise your self-talks and choose another emotional response. On the bottom half of your worksheet, in the left hand column, write down the same event. Then, work your way across the six categories, revising the old self-talks and writing new, more positive alternatives. You may need to refer back to the preceding section of this chapter and review the material on each of the self-talks and how to revise them. In the D1 column, reframe your demands into more flexible wants and preferences. In the D2 column, reduce your denial. Accept what has happened and begin to develop some insight. In the 0 column rid yourself of the awful over-evaluation of the event as terrible or horrible, and begin to formulate more realistic and accurate evaluations of the event. Then, under AN1, create a more objective picture of future developments and note what you can do to start making things better right now. Under AN2, discard the absolute evaluations of yourself, others, and the situation; look for positive attributes that can be built upon. Finally, discard the unrealistic mind reading and compose more realistic self-talks about the perceptions and thoughts of others.

When you have written down the new, coping self-talks in all six categories, read them over several times. At first they may seem quite different and hard to believe compared to the habitual, stress-producing self-talks that you are so accustomed to repeating inwardly. Using these new self-talks to evaluate the event, move on to the emotional response column. List your feelings and rate their intensity. Write down your physiological reactions and behavior. It is likely that you will notice a significant change in your emotional response. Strong negative feelings may well be reduced in intensity or disappear altogether. More adaptive feelings may arise, such as concern and interest instead of fear and anxiety. Physiological reactions may be much milder, and you may feel inclined to actions that will solve problems rather than create them.

The crucial point is that by changing our self-talks we can create a healthier and more constructive emotional response. Revising our self-talks is a very effective way to reduce the stress resulting from excessive emotional responding. And the resultant healthy thinking is like a skill that we become better at the more we practice. This written exercise provides good practice. Typically, if we do this written procedure once or twice we can become proficient at changing our self-talks on an ongoing basis. Whenever we note a dysfunctional emotional reaction we can look for and revise the self-talks that create the problem. Working with the self-talks, our mental content gives us a very practical and effective means for accessing the mental factors that create and maintain stress. As mentioned earlier in the chapter, there are also two other dimensions of the mind that figure in the stress equation. These are the dimensions of mental process and mental structure. Let us now consider the mental processes that influence our stress levels.

Mental Process and Inner Dynamics

As we gain experience in analyzing our self-talks, we may note that certain patterns seem to come up again and again. It is as if we are predisposed toward certain self-talks and emotional responses. For example we may find that we continually get caught up in overreacting to events and then feel tense and anxious. Or we may notice a tendency to engage in always-never thinking and find ourselves feeling depressed and hopeless. It seems that these predispositions are maintained by deep and enduring mental processes that profoundly and consistently influence our reactions to inner and outer events. Ultimately then, to master our emotions and to prevent stress we must come to understand and then work with these deeper mental dynamics. Along these lines, the ancient tradition of yoga presents an analysis of mental processes that is clear and understandable and will lead to many practical approaches for change. In this tradition, five sources of suffering are listed. These five sources, or *kleshas* as they are called in Sanskrit, are the causes of mental, emotional, and physical suffering. In modern parlance we could say that they are the root causes of stress. These kleshas are identified in the second chapter of the *Yoga Sutras* of Patanjali, one of the basic resource books of yoga science.[7] The five kleshas are described as the absence of knowledge, false identification, attachment, aversion, and clinging to life.

All of the following four kleshas really arise from the first one—the absence of true knowledge. More specifically, this lack of knowledge is ignorance of our true nature and of our place and role in life. Without this knowledge, the principle of false identification, the second klesha, comes into play as we seek out various identifications and cling to them. Then, from these assumed identities we become attracted to objects that we subjectively find pleasing and avoid objects and experiences that we find aversive. This creates a world of positive and negative attachments and describes the action of the third and fourth kleshas. Finally, we become so involved in our self-created world of identities, attachments, and aversions that we are reluctant to give it up. This is the fifth klesha, clinging to life.

Before we discuss these kleshas in detail and describe methods for alleviating the suffering and stress that arise from each, we can illustrate the operation of the kleshas through the following hypothetical situation: a businessman is attending a convention in a city far away from his home town. In between meetings he decides to go for a walk. Unfortunately, a mugger sneaks up on him, knocks him unconscious, and steals his wallet. When he wakes up he has total amnesia and has no idea of who he is. He is picked up by the police, and as he listens to their descriptions he hears that he is a male of average height, and has certain physical features. He begins to identify himself according to their description. After some time the court gives him a new name, Roger Doe, and a social security number. An employment office finds him a job as a carpenter's helper. Now his new identity is taking shape and on the basis of this identity, he begins to develop patterns of likes and dislikes. He becomes attached to those experiences and objects that enhance his new identity, even as he avoids those things that threaten or demean his new identity. He develops an entire matrix of pleasure and pain attachments. And of course these attachments are accompanied by a whole range of emotions. He has positive feelings when he obtains what is pleasurable and negative feelings when he experiences something painful.

One day on the street someone who knew him before his accident recognizes him. This person calls out and tries to remind Roger of who he really is. But Roger doesn't want to hear it; he becomes afraid and runs away. He doesn't want to give up his new identity. Roger's fear grows and he becomes wary of going out in public places where someone might recognize him.

Roger's potential for suffering corresponds to the kleshas. His original problem began when he became

ignorant of his true identity. The plot thickened when he
assumed a new identity and from this perspective developed a world of pleasure and pain attachments. Finally he
began to cling to his assumed identity and fear any change.
From the perspective of yoga, we all create suffering in a
similar manner. Deep within our psyche the operation of
these kleshas predisposes us to a disturbed mind which
leads to emotional upset, with the end result of suffering
and stress. Consequently, to calm the mind and overcome
stress we need a program to deal with each of these kleshas.

Let us begin by considering some ways to resolve the
fifth klesha, clinging to life. It is said in the Yoga Sutras
that even the educated have this strong feeling of clinging
to life and fear of annihilation of the self.[8] This fear of
death is a very powerful emotion that creates anxiety and
stirs up the mind. However, in the tradition of yoga, death
is viewed as a transition, and life is filled with transitions.
From this perspective life is a series of deaths and rebirths
and constant transitions. We give up one way of being and
grow into another. We give up the pleasures of adolescence
for the more meaningful satisfactions of adulthood. Interestingly, the relaxation pose in yoga is called *shavasana*
and it means the corpse pose.[9] In shavasana we lie down in
a state of tension, let go of the holding, and are reborn in a
relaxed state and feel refreshed.

If we study the nature of life and see the constant and
healthful action of transitions we can begin to overcome
our basic fear and clinging to life. We can begin to cultivate
a philosophy of welcoming change and transition as the
necessary concomitants of growth and well-being. We can
come to feel and believe that there is nothing to fear. We
can feel comfortable with life, secure in our sense of self
and open to transition.

The fifth klesha tends to operate as an underlying and
pervasive anxiety of which we are seldom fully aware. Only
occasionally does an awareness of our clinging and fear of

change emerge into our consciousness.

But the third and fourth kleshas, the forces of attraction and aversion play a significant role in our conscious experience. Our attraction to pleasure and our aversion to pain create emotional turmoil. Our attachments are often the source of the rigid demands that we make of others, ourselves, and life in general. When our demands are thwarted, we experience a surge of negative emotions. These negative emotions, when experienced too frequently and to intensely, create stress.

Yoga teaches that the way to overcome attraction and aversion is to cultivate non-attachment and dispassion. This is accomplished by developing a deep and abiding attitude of equanimity toward the events and objects in our environment. This idea of inner peace and balance is described in many ancient texts. One of the clearest statements is found in the Bhagavad Gita, where the great teacher Krishna provides his student, Arjuna, with the following instruction on the topic of emotional balance:

> For the pleasures that come from the world bear in them sorrows to come. They come and go, they are transient: not in them do the wise find joy. But he who on the earth, before his departure, can endure the storms of desire and wrath, this man is a Yogi, this man has joy.
>
> He has an inner joy, he has inner gladness, and he has found inner Light. This Yogi attains the Nirvana of Brahman: he is one with God and goes unto God.[10]

This passage illustrates the transitory nature of pleasure and pain. A consideration of daily life indeed demonstrates the fleeting and ever changing nature of pleasure and pain. For example, we may experience a gourmet meal as the height of pleasure and yet even as we are finishing our dessert, other thoughts come crowding in. We may begin to worry about how we can have an even better meal in the future. Attachment to pleasure is like an addiction; we continually seek higher and higher levels of pleasure to satisfy our needs. Yet even the greatest of pleasure can be diminished as we worry about our financial affairs, argue with someone, or even suffer from indigestion. And in a similar vein even sorrow is transitory. In the midst of grief or sadness we may be surprised to notice some small pleasure in the events of daily life. Thus feelings of both pleasure and pain are essentially shifting and impermanent.

Rather than becoming attached to the sensation of pleasure and trying to hold on to it while pushing pain away, it is far better simply to observe and witness these feelings, avoiding the internal judging process by which we overreact to pleasure and pain. Instead we can observe and take note of the experience, watch its development and its passing with an even, dispassionate interest.

Two points concerning the nature of the pleasure and pain that we have in the world are emphasized again and again in the tradition of yoga: the objects of the world are transitory and can never give us full satisfaction. We always end up seeking more pleasure, and attempting to guarantee the pleasures we have. In a similar fashion, we put increasing effort into avoiding pain and trying to prevent it from coming into our life. Yoga recommends dispassion and nonattachment as a method for dealing with pleasure and pain.

Sometimes, however, people become confused about the idea of non-attachment. They mistakenly think that non-attachment means to reject and scorn the activities, objects, and experiences of the world. They develop an unhealthy and phony asceticism and deny themselves material possessions, while harboring anger toward those who have them. The material objects themselves are not the problem; it is our attitude toward them, our attachment, that is the problem. Yoga encourages a healthy attitude toward material objects. We are encouraged to enjoy the experience and to utilize material objects to accomplish our goals, but to avoid becoming attached to them.

Non-attachment is also built upon inner experience. For example, when we have a fulfilling inner experience we feel a reduced need to seek fulfillment from the objects and experiences of the world. The science of yoga is a route to the fulfilling inner experience of peace and contentment, and involves a progression from a relaxation of the body, nervous system, and mind to a realization of one's own nature.

We usually seek to know ourselves and measure our value based on our external accomplishments and material acquisitions. As a result, there is considerable drive behind our attachments. Yoga science is based on the idea that we have another avenue for affirming our personal reality. Inner exploration and self-awareness can allow us to feel real and complete from within, and as we begin to experience this satisfying inner knowledge of ourself our attachments to external sources of self-affirmation are weakened. Then the possibilities for a healthy non-attachment grow. When we feel complete within, we don't need external accomplishments and objects in the same way. We are free to express ourselves through possessions and deeds, but we are not dependent upon them.

Our desires and attachments are organized in relation to who we think we should be or who we want to be. Therefore, the practice of non-attachment leads us to consider issues of who we really are. These considerations bring us face to face with the second klesha, or source of suffering: the problem of false identification. We readily become engaged in a struggle to maintain our assumed identities. This struggle is the source of considerable inner tension and stress. Maurice Nicoll, who has written extensively on self-development within the Gurdjieff tradition, aptly describes the inner struggle that results from protecting our assumed identities:

A man must become quite open to himself without deception. This is true relaxation. He must cease to hold in himself certain beliefs about himself. Anxiety and fear, which prevent us from relaxing, subtly arise when a man endeavors to maintain what is not really himself. He lives on one side of himself. The False Personality, always preoccupied with different forms of internal considering, with questions of whether a good impression is being made and appearances kept up, causes a strain in being. It is as if a man kept standing on his toes and did not understand why he felt exhausted. All the time he is keeping something up which is not himself—something imaginary—something which does not fit him. And this happens with everyone. If we had no False Personality all this anxiety and nervousness which all secretly feel about themselves, whether they admit it or not, would vanish. Not only would relationships to others change, but our relationship to ourselves. We then would understand what it is to relax.[11]

True relaxation and mastery of stress cannot occur as long as we are struggling to maintain a certain view of ourself and to outwardly present that view. This insecurity about who we are creates a great deal of anxiety. Due to this anxiety we develop defense mechanisms and try to suppress certain parts of ourself and to promote the other parts. It is important, then, to deal with the issue of false identification—to become comfortable with ourself and to transcend inner doubt and anxiety. One way to work with this second klesha is to cultivate self-acceptance by adjusting our self-talks, particularly our self-demands and self-condemnations. If we engage in these types of self-talks we are feeding the fire of false identification, adding more tension and self-blame. We can relieve this tension by beginning to accept ourself without judgements and criteria.

From the perspective of yoga, self-acceptance is a dynamic process. Love and compassion start with our self-appraisal. Self-acceptance is based on balanced self-observation. We observe our qualities, both the things we like and the things we don't like, without judging them. We are open to change but free from anger and disgust. As we develop greater self-acceptance we avoid creating guilt and tension, and we can acknowledge aspects of ourself without fear and anxiety.

In fact, one of the most destructive aspects of the identification process is that we expend a great deal of energy reinforcing and promoting parts of ourself that we like, and hiding and suppressing aspects of ourself that we dislike. In our social interactions we strive to project a certain identity, while inwardly we struggle to hide unliked aspects. As Swami Rama writes, "A teacher keenly observes the behavior of his students, and he finds that many students do not have respect for themselves. Instead they condemn themselves and try to hide the unwanted parts of their personalities by creating masks for themselves. The images they present to others are based on their insecurities. That is unhealthy and hinders the growth of the student. A good student is aware of and reveres his real Self, and he practices maintaining constant consciousness of the center within. That is real self-respect, and if one loses it, he becomes the victim of vanity and creates defense mechanisms."[12]

Loosening the process of identification and gaining a true self-acceptance allows us to become much more flexible. It actually leads toward personality integration. In our relations with others, we can be more truly responsive when we are free from the feeling that we have to project a certain way of being. We are then able to move in and out of identities with greater dexterity. We can be a child among children, a business person in the business world, a friend among friends, a lover with our life partner, and a

teacher before students. We can move gracefully from
identity to identity as need and purpose dictate. Simultaneously we can be open to all aspects of ourself and draw
energy and creativity from those parts that we may have
previously hidden or suppressed.

Identities, in and of themselves, do not produce suffering. It is our insecurity and our clinging to these identities that create the suffering. When we practice non-
judgmental self-observation and self-acceptance, we can
overcome these negative effects. Then we can use our
identities in a creative sense. They become instruments for
the expression of our growth rather than shackles that hold
us back.

Ultimately, in order to deal with the issue of false
identification we must come face to face with the first
klesha, ignorance of our true nature. This ignorance acts as
the most fundamental cause of suffering and stress. Without knowledge of our true identity we continually become
embroiled in the search to create and the struggle to
maintain and protect false identities. Each identity, in turn,
becomes the breeding ground for attachment and we then
cling to the world of painful experience that we have
created. The ancient texts of yoga were very clear in
pointing out that knowledge of our true identity is crucial
for liberation from suffering and the achievement of maximal health. In his commentary on the *Yoga Sutras,* Pandit
Arya presents the following quotation taken from the *Bhaga-
vata-purana*: "Liberation means to abandon the state as
though one were some other, and to dwell in the identity of
one's own nature."[13]

Within the tradition of yoga there are a number of
methods of obtaining the knowledge and experience of
one's true identity. Some of these methods have become
separate systems of yoga. For example, there is *jnana* yoga,
in which intellectual study, reasoning, and deduction are
utilized to overcome the limits of false identification and to

establish awareness of one's true nature. There is also the path of *karma* yoga, the yoga of action, in which one focuses on serving others and giving to humanity as a means to overcome narrow ego identifications. Or there is the path of *bhakti* yoga, through which one transcends suffering through love and devotion to a personal deity. These various paths are well-suited to certain individual temperaments and each person may find a system of yoga that is most compatible with his or her effort to establish a true sense of self.

One method for establishing true self-awareness that is common to all paths is meditation. Meditation allows for a letting go of the false, assumed identities and an emergence of our true nature. Often, in the tradition of yoga, a distinction is made between self and Self. When written in lower case, "self" refers to our assumed identities, and when capitalized, "Self" refers to our essential nature and true identity. As defined by Swami Rama, "The Self is eternal and its essential nature is existence, consciousness, and bliss. It permeates the waking, dreaming, and deep sleep states and remains above all mundane pains and pleasures."[14] Meditation is a direct method for obtaining awareness of this greater Self. During meditation we are able to quiet the mind, let go of the thoughts associated with attachments and assumed identities, and begin to simply and quietly experience our true nature. This experience allows us to rise above suffering and to eliminate stress.

Those underlying dynamics create suffering in our life and predispose us to engage in stress-producing self-talks. Overcoming these five sources of suffering is not an easy process. There are increasingly subtle layers of attachments and identifications, so that when we rid ourself of one set of attachments we encounter yet another. The same is true for our identities. Accordingly, we can avail ourselves again and again of every opportunity that helps us to loosen our attachments, integrate our personality, and come into increasing contact with our true Self. With efforts underway to overcome the kleshas and with a growing ability to recognize and transform stress-producing self-talks, we are ready to examine still another dimension of the mind that figures in the stress equation. This dimension is the structure or state of the mind itself.

The Structure of the Mind

In the tradition of yoga there is a principle that mind has a certain structure that changes according to our mental and emotional state. Mind is seen as an energy field. When the field is scattered and dispersed there is little strength in the field. When the mind is distracted and tense, filled with worries and conflicts, then the field of mind is scattered and weak. This is a stressful state. We experience it subjectively as an inability to concentrate, while the mind races from thought to thought. When the mind is in this state, we are more likely to make errors, forget things, and to be indecisive, all of which can feed the cycle of stress. On the other hand, when the field of mind is collected and focused there is a feeling of inner mastery and an ability to concentrate effectively on challenges in the environment. The focused and cohesive mind field is healthy, while the scattered and distracted mind is stressful.

In yoga science, five descriptors are used to describe the general condition of the mind. These five span the continuum from least healthy to most healthy. These five descriptors are "disturbed," "somnolent/stupefied," "distracted," "one-pointed," and "controlled."[15] The goal of yoga is to overcome the first three conditions, to achieve gradual mastery of the one-pointed mind, and finally to fully control the thought waves, so that true wisdom and Self-awareness may arise. Learning to overcome the three lower conditions and to concentrate the mind is a crucial process in achieving health. Many of the practices of yoga are performed so that the mind can be made more one-pointed. For example, during hatha yoga stretching or breathing exercises, one should focus attention on those activities and thereby achieve a one-pointed mind.

There are, however, a number of other techniques in yoga that have as their primary goal making the mind one-pointed. These are concentration techniques that are an essential part of the yogic program for self-improvement. One such technique is to focus the attention on the breath. The breath is an ideal object of concentration because it moves, changes, and has a rhythm. The mind can more easily move from its scattered state to focus on something as interesting and rhythmic as the breath.

Specifically, one can observe the rhythm of exhalation and inhalation, notice the movement of the abdominal muscles, or attend to the sensation of the breath as it flows in and out of the nostrils. Typically, the air feels slightly cooler and drier as it flows in, and warmer and more moist as it flows out. In another exercise, one might simply "count" inhalations and exhalations, counting forward and backward from one to some number. Even five minutes of these techniques will have a dramatic effect. The mind will feel rested, refreshed, and relaxed. There is also a feeling of joy and contentment that accompanies concentration. We may be familiar with this feeling while deeply engrossed in a book or engaged in some type of work with our hands. In the case of the yogic concentration exercises, the concentration is not dependent on some external activity and the effects are greater.

There are other methods for concentration that emphasize one or more of the sensory pathways. For example, there is a concentration exercise known as *trataka* or gazing.[16] This exercise is performed by focusing the eyes on either a part of the body or an external object. For example, one can gaze at a candle flame or a dot placed at eye level at a comfortable distance of two to three feet. In the beginning, even a few minutes of this exercise is quite helpful in terms of concentrating the mind. As one's capacity grows the length of the exercise can be extended. Gazing is reputed to improve the eyes, cleanse the mind, and strengthen the ability to concentrate. The ultimate effect is to calm and settle the mind and make it a more effective instrument.

Another form of concentration involves focusing on sounds. Here, one imagines being at the center of a great circle. Then one listens to the various sounds in the environment and notes where they come from in the circle. Some of the sounds may be steady, as from a furnace or a clock, and some may be transient, as a car passes by, or as someone opens and closes a door. The point is to concentrate gently on the various sounds. As with the other exercises, the goal is to focus the mind. As that focusing occurs, the mind field is transformed from scattered, dispersed, and weak into centered, balanced, and strong. One feels an inner peace and sees the world with greater clarity.

The manner in which concentration is performed is very important. Proper concentration should have a gentle, easy, and restful quality about it. It is useful to prepare for concentration by letting go of external involvements, relaxing the muscles, and steadying the breath. As we begin to focus the mind we may observe its tendency to wander and jump from theme to theme and to be distracted by bodily sensations. Such digressions and distractions are quite common. We simply work within our capacity and guide the mind back to the object of concentration. The mind is, in fact, quite trainable and with regular and persistent effort we can make surprising strides in our ability to achieve and maintain concentration.

In the *Yoga Sutras,* "concentration" is defined as the confinement of the mind to one place.[17] Such confinement is not to be thought of as a harsh incarceration that creates resistance, but a loving training process like taming a wild horse to be a useful helper and a good friend. In the yoga system, concentration is considered to be the first internal step on the path of self-transformation. It is the foundation for refining the mind and transforming the personality. It is a powerful approach for reducing mental stress and enhancing the health and effectiveness of the mind. Practicing concentration for five to fifteen minutes from one to three times a day can be quite helpful.

Summary

We have discussed the crucial role of the mind in controlling the stress response. The mind both initiates the stress response and presents an opportunity to reduce and regulate this response. We have examined three dimensions of mind that can be worked with to reduce and ultimately prevent stress. These are mental content, mental dynamics, and mental structure. Stress producing, habitual patterns in all three of these dimensions can be resistant to change. Yet the benefits in terms of reduced stress, greater effectiveness, and enhanced health are so great that it is worth the effort to begin to make changes at the mental level.

Change at the mental level is a process. We must commit ourselves to the introspection and concentration that, when properly conducted, inevitably create healthful change in our mental patterns. Of all the objects in the world, we are able to have the most control over our mind. In the words of the Buddha, "It is wrong to think that misfortunes come from the East or from the West; they originate within one's own mind. Therefore, it is foolish to guard against misfortunes from the external world and leave the inner mind uncontrolled."[18]

CHAPTER 6

Fear, Stress, and the Quality of Life

Phil Nuernberger, Ph.D.

The quality of our daily life definitely influences our stress levels. The quality of our life is in turn influenced by our persistent underlying emotional patterns. All too often our concerns regarding the quality of life do not address this internal emotional level but instead are directed solely toward the external material world. Consequently, we may come to equate the quality of life with such factors as noise level, air pollution, the number of cultural events and institutions in our area, the availability of public transportation, the number of parks, the prevailing weather patterns, the opportunities for shopping, and even the crime rate: if all of these factors are positive, we expect that the quality of life will be excellent and that stress levels will be lower.

Actually, the phrase "the quality of life" may have many different meanings to different people. We can optimally understand it as the attempt to achieve excellence in living, an attempt to enrich and enjoy life to the greatest possible extent. In one very positive sense, it is a manifestation of

This chapter is based on an earlier article that appeared by the same title in Dawn *magazine, Volume 2, Number 2, 1982.*

man's curiosity, and expression of the desire for higher knowledge. Seeking this quality of life has, unfortunately, also been pretty much of a failure. In all honesty, we must admit that the "great mass of men" still lead lives of (not necessarily quiet) desperation. We have only been able to achieve more sophisticated forms of distraction (e.g., the widespread and extensive use of television) than we had in earlier years. It is not that the search for quality in life is a will-o'-the-wisp, an empty gesture which can never be achieved. Rather, the error is in the focus of our search. We fully expect some "thing" to bring us everlasting joy and happiness. New cars, a more "meaningful" play or work of art, the development of "more satisfying" relationships, the acquisition of degrees and letters of honor after one's name, even the desperate grabbing on and clinging to a religious belief or symbol, are all touted as "the one way," as the answer to life's ills and spills.

Yet underneath it all, our fears eat away in our hearts, bringing us imbalance, pain and death—not only the death of the body, a condition through which all must pass, but also the day-to-day little deaths of our joy, our contentment, our peace. It is our fears that rob us, that sneak in dark places and steal the excellence from our life. It is our fears that hold and prevent us from enjoying that which we have already and that which we will have. It is our fears, both large and small, that keep us from the experience of the simplicity and joy of life. And it is our fears that we *must* conquer if we are to attain the excellence that is our birthright. The search for the quality of life can be successful only to the extent that we come to understand and conquer fear.

What is this dragon called fear? Upon analysis we come to find that fear is really the anticipation of loss or harm to one's sense of "I"-ness, or yogic ego. This loss or harm may be physical, but more often it is social or psychological. It may involve the person himself, or objects to which he is emotionally attached or with which he is identified, such as his family, friends, football team, house, job, position in society, reputation, and so on. A key point is the *perceived* (consciously or unconsciously) *probability* of loss or pain. It is this uncertainty tied with expectation that allows for the development of the "what if" syndrome, which contributes to fear. It is important to see that when probability becomes actuality, fear becomes transformed into depression, or anger, or even relief. Fear only exists within the confines of anticipation; it cannot exist within the direct experience of the event itself. Thus, while one can experience fear, the fear itself is ephemeral; it disappears when the actual event that was feared takes place.

Memory also plays a key role in the experience of fear. The anticipation of harm must necessarily be based on some past experience; there must be some memory of pain that is recalled and projected into the future. That is, the perception of events occurring now is interpreted as painful because of a past similar experience that resulted in some kind of harm (pain, loss). This impact (interpretive framework) of memory is nearly always on the unconscious level, which only facilitates and strengthens the perceptual habit. The power of past experience is more easily seen if one watches the development and growth of a child: as the child accumulates experiences, he begins to develop fears. (This is a complex process in which the parents play a significant role. The point, however, is that by having painful experiences, which are unavoidable in life, and thus having memory traces of such experiences, the child develops the potential for fear.) Thus, we can see that fear has something to do with the past (memory) and the future (anticipation), but it does not really exist in the present. As we shall see later, it is this peculiar time-dependent aspect of fear that provides for the control and eventual elimination of fear.

There is another aspect of fear that is not clearly

understood; that is, the common tendency to confuse the experience of fear, which is an emotional response, with the perception of danger or harm, which is a discrimination of cause/effect relationships. While the emotion of fear requires the perception of danger (harm or loss), it is very possible to perceive danger without becoming fearful. In fact, the emotion of fear can distort the perceptual process, possibly leading to even greater danger. Thus, we must understand that particular factor which differentiates the emotion of fear from the discrimination of danger and the motivation to protect oneself.

The motivation to protect oneself (and those objects in the world with which one is emotionally identified) is found in the primitive urge of self-preservation. This primitive urge or drive, like the other three primitive urges of food, sleep, and sex, is a natural part of the biological organism. In yoga, these urges are often referred to as fountains because they are a channeling of energy. The urge for self-preservation is a channeling of energy to protect not only the physical existence but also the psychological existence of the individual. These two are the fundamental framework of the yogic ego, ahankara, or sense of "I"-ness. This flow of energy is not an emotion, or fear itself; rather, it is the energy that underlies the emotion.

While the emotional energy is provided by this primitive urge, according to yoga the focusing and utilization of this energy is the task of the four functions of the mind: *manas, chitta, ahankara,* and *buddhi.* Briefly, it is the function of manas to collect and organize sensory data. It is the function of chitta to provide the experiential background, or memory, by which the sensory data is organized and interpreted (i.e., given meaning). Ahankara, the yogic ego or sense of "I"-ness, provides a center or identity that is the agent and/or recipient of the action. The function of buddhi, the discriminative faculty, is to recognize and determine cause/effect relationships.

Thus it is the functions of mind that channel and direct the energy from the primitive urge into appropriate action. The following example will illustrate how this happens. Let's say that you are taking a hike. You come to a fence, climb over, and start across an open field. Suddenly you see a large four-legged animal with horns on its head running toward you (all of your perceptions are due to the functioning of *manas*). You immediately recognize that it is a bull (a function of *chitta*, or memory). You also recognize that this bull is on a collision course (a function of *buddhi*, discrimination) with *you* (a function of *ahankara*, the sense of "I"-ness). Your adrenalin flows, your heart pumps faster, and you immediately run and vault right over the fence (energy supplied by the primitive urge). Now you may or may not have felt fear (the bull was far away, the fence was close), but you certainly had the energy to run, jump, and protect yourself. In short, you had the ability to enter a state of arousal. Actually, you may even feel fear after the event has passed.

Thus we can see that perception, memory, ego or sense of "I"-ness, and discrimination, supported by and guiding the motivational energy (experienced as arousal), are all necessary aspects of the process of the discrimination of danger and the self-preservation response. Yet this is still not the emotion of fear. It is possible to experience this energy flow directed toward self-protection, and to take the actions necessary to protect oneself, without experiencing any fear. To understand fear, we must understand the nature of emotions. We see that emotional energy flows from the four primitive fountains of food, sex, sleep, and self-preservation. To satisfy these urges, we select certain objects from our environment. For example, to satisfy my need for food, I may choose an apple or a piece of cherry pie. To satisfy my need for self-preservation, I may do exercises to build my vital capacities. I may buy a Cadillac to build my ego. This focusing of energy to obtain a specific object (or to avoid a specific object that is associated with pain) is the level of desire. Thus, when I become hungry, I begin to think of specific objects that I think will protect or enhance my ego or my physical/psychological/social existence.

The bond between the object and the flow of energy is created by experiencing pleasure or pain as the object is obtained. This bond, or connection, between the object and the energy flow can become so strong as to appear to be inseparable. Thus the desire (or flow of energy) and the object of the desire come to be seen as one thing. This can completely conceal the fact that there are other objects (or courses of action) that could satisfy the desire (to feel satisfied, complete, happy, secure, etc.). It is this dependency upon the object of the desire that creates the emotional response. If we are dependent upon the object to satisfy our needs and we are unable to obtain that object (or series of actions) and thus satisfy our desire, the result is a negative emotion. The emotion is negative because it creates a physical and psychological imbalance. Fear is that negative emotion that is rooted in our dependency upon those objects that satisfy the desires springing from our urge for self-preservation. Not only does fear create imbalance, but this imbalance leads to psychological and physical conditions that interfere with the discriminative process (which is vital if one is to accurately perceive danger and the ways to avoid it). Fear can also bring about the very events that one fears, that is, it can act as a self-fulfilling prophecy. We can now begin to see that fear, a negative emotion, is not only unnecesary for self-protection, but in many ways actually leads to even greater danger.

We now understand two key aspects of fear, which can help us to gain control over this emotion. The first is the recognition that fear exists only in the anticipation of an event and cannot exist in the immediacy of the experience itself, in the here-and-now. Secondly, the emotion of fear is necessarily rooted in our dependency upon the objects of those desires arising from the primitive urge of self-preservation. Implicit in this dependency is our inability to discriminate between the desire and the object of the desire, thus preventing us from utilizing any number of possible alternative objects by which to satisfy the desire. Our goal, of course, is to become fearless, to control and eventually eliminate fear from our lives. This becomes possible if we learn to control the mind's tendency to anticipate, and if we begin to understand our proper relationship to the objects in our lives.

If we study ourselves and others, and if we examine our experiences, we will come to know that meditation is the only process that can lead the mind to be centered in the immediate present and not to wander into useless anticipation or expectation. When the time aspect of mind is thus controlled, we no longer can be fearful. The meditative form most directly relevant to our daily living is meditation in action. This is the form of meditation that develops perceptual purity: the ability to see without being influenced by memory or past experience. This is the ability "to be as a child in the world," to see every moment as a new and unique moment. The yogic practice of breath awareness is an important tool in this form of meditative process.

But also necessary is the ability to free ourselves from dependency upon the objects of the world, to be able to differentiate desire from objects, and to have the freedom to choose. This is only possible when one is able to calm the body and mind and experience directly that superconscious state that is complete in and of itself, that is free from all attachments or dependency on the objects of the world. This is the experience of enlightenment, the universal consciousness characterized by completeness, bliss, and tranquility. It is this experience of an identity or Self that is free from all disturbances which will also free one from all fears. This is the goal of concentrative meditation which, through one-pointed concentration, can pierce the deeper aspects of mind to reach a state of pure awareness. Freedom from fear is a natural consequence of this experience of pure consciousness.

The study of yoga, the comprehensive science of consciousness is a systematic way to free oneself from fear. There are a number of steps to yoga which require our full participation and effort, for without the direct experience that is provided by the regular practice of meditation, there is no freedom from fear. Thus, the quality of life does not depend on some thing in our world, but on ourselves. It is the freedom from fear that will allow us to live with quality, to achieve the excellence in life which is our birthright. No government, no job or position in society, no amount of money, no preacher, no savior can give inner peace. Only when we master our fears will we come to know the pure joy of life itself. It is up to us.

CHAPTER 7

Meditation and the Quiet Mind

John R. Harvey, Ph.D.

Of all the techniques available for managing stress, meditation is surely the finest. It operates at the most subtle level of stress causation, the realm of the mind. Stress is an emotional response that arises in the activity of both the conscious and unconscious dimensions of the mind—it is a result of the way we perceive and think. Accordingly, the degree of our underlying mental attachments determines the intensity and duration of the emotional response that we call stress. When the mind is quiet, balanced, and open—as during the state of true meditation—it is impossible to experience stress.

Thus, it is worthwhile to consider what meditation is and to become aware of what it is not. Meditation is an inner method for working with the mind. It is not a religious practice. Meditation involves applying a series of systematic steps to produce certain desirable and helpful changes in one's state of consciousness. It is not a way to see vivid colors, have intense sensory experiences, or get "high." Meditation is a method whereby we become fully acquainted with ourselves in an independent and self-reliant manner. It is not self-hypnosis, nor is it in any way based on suggestion.

Meditation is a way to free the mind from disturbing thoughts—a practical method that can be used in everyday life. It does not demand that a person in any way "drop out," change his style of clothing, eat weird food, or join a cult. In fact, such dramatic external changes may merely create disturbances in the mind or disruptions in daily life, and may be the antithesis of a sincere, meaningful, meditative process of change.

It may be most useful to consider meditation as a procedure for working with the mind. Just as there are exercises and techniques for toning and cleansing the body and procedures for using the breath to relax and balance the nervous system, so also does meditation involve using a definite set of procedures to create a state of mind that is free of stress.

Meditation is a method for working with all the levels of mind by first exploring and then guiding the transformation of both the content and the structure of the mind. And meditation also has other implications, as it leads to the expansion of the personality and the clarification of our purpose in life.

Meditation as described here is distinct from the common meaning of meditation as a process of pondering or ruminating on some topic. "Meditation" is the English equivalent for the Sanskrit word *dhyana*. This term is clearly and very specifically defined in a number of classical yoga texts. The ancient yogis, who were interested in methods to overcome suffering and achieve self-development, carefully systematized, studied, and described the practice of meditation.

One of the clearest descriptions of meditation can be found in the *Yoga Sutras of Patanjali*, a classical text on yoga practices.[1] The meditative process includes three phases. The first phase of meditation might actually be more accurately called concentration. It involves fixing the attention upon and confining the mind to one object.

The next phase, which is more properly meditation, involves establishing an unbroken mental "flow" toward the object of meditation. The phrase "object of meditation" means any image, word, or concept used as a point of concentration for the mind.

This stands in clear contrast to the mind's usual habit of haphazardly racing from one thought to the other. Meditation is a total focus upon one object. It is a stable, uniform flow of the mind that is untouched by distracting or disturbing thoughts, and it produces a profound experience of serenity.

The third phase of meditation is somewhat more difficult to grasp, as it is beyond our everyday experience. This phase involves total absorption, in which we go beyond thought, empty the mind, and then experientially apprehend the real nature of the designated object of meditation. This is an experience of illumination. In summary, then, the process of meditation includes concentrating the mind, establishing an unbroken and continuous flow, and then experiencing absorption.

There are a great number of meditative techniques, which vary according to the object of meditation. For example, a beginning meditative technique in the Zen tradition involves resting the mind on the flow of the breath, counting the exhalations up to ten, and then continually repeating this procedure. For many people, this is an ideal technique with which to begin, because the breath has a definite rhythm and because counting is also a concrete task to occupy the mind. And as a deep, continuous mental flow is established, we may experience the unique consciousness of meditation.

In the tradition of yoga, specific words are also given as the focal object of meditation. These are called mantras, and are combinations of syllables or words, designed to be compact versions or "seeds" of a balanced state of consciousness. The meditator not only steadies the mind on the sound of the mantra as it is repeated inwardly, but also eventually, at the stage of absorption in the mantra, comes to realize its full meaning and experience. The continual repetition of the mantra then helps to bring forward the creative inner potentials and beneficial characteristics of the meditator.

Some mantras are suitable for anyone beginning to practice meditation. Others may be given by a teacher because the mantra fits the needs and potentials of a specific student. There is, in fact, an entire, intricate science of mantras that is well beyond the scope of our discussion.* Suffice it to say that mantra meditation is a definite and carefully developed approach to the practice of meditation.

Several techniques should be mentioned. For example, we may focus our attention on a specific center or point in the body, or we may meditate upon a geometric pattern known as a yantra. These are more subtle techniques and typically require the guidance of a skilled teacher. There is even a technique in which there is no object or focus. The meditator merely opens the mind and dispassionately watches the mental content and process until it eventually quiets down and the mind is still.

The variety of meditative methods accommodates the variety of character types and personality styles present in human beings, so that there is a technique of meditation that is appropriate for almost everyone. Whatever the method used, the key point is to begin to experience and regularly practice meditation.

The systematic establishment of the meditative state has a number of important effects on stress. Meditation serves as the perfect antidote for, or counterbalance to, the

---

*Footnote: For more detailed information on the science of mantra, the interested reader should consult *Mantra and Meditation* by Usharbudh Arya, D.Litt. (Honesdale, Pennsylvania, Himalayan Publishers, 1981).

stress in our lives. When we experience stress, the mind typically is racing from topic to topic. For example, we may think, in rapid succession, about what we need to do in the future, events of the past, or what we are doing in the present. The mind becomes exhausted by running from topic to topic in this manner. In meditation, by contrast, the mind rests on one object.

Actually, as tiring as this process of leaping from thought to thought is, the most crucial aspect is that there is an emotional charge coupled with each thought: feelings of frustration and anxiety may accompany our thoughts about the things we need to do, guilt and sadness may color each memory of past events, or anger and pressure may be connected with our current activity.

It is this instant flow of emotional responses triggered by our racing thoughts that acts to set off, maintain, and exacerbate the physiological activation of stress. From the perspective of meditation, these emotional charges that accompany our thoughts are known as attachments, and it is attachments that create stress.

As we progress into the meditative state we become increasingly free of these emotionally charged attachments because we increasingly experience a state of inner peace and joy that is unrelated to these experiences of pleasure and pain. There is a crucial process in meditation called "witnessing" that allows us to do this by leading to non-attachment.

When thoughts and issues come up in the mind during meditation we simply witness or observe them without further reaction or rumination. This is in contrast to our usual pattern of ruminating on our negative feelings, strengthening them, and even adding new negative feelings—for example, feeling angry with ourselves for becoming sad or becoming still more anxious about being anxious.

On the other hand, when we observe our thoughts without reacting, these thoughts slow down and such feelings subside. Then the entire pattern of physiological stress declines. This, indeed, is managing stress at the most internal level. This does not mean that issues in the external world, which we often call "stressors," in any way vanish. What it means is that we have the opportunity to exercise much greater choice in how we respond to these various demands and challenges.

While meditating, we simply observe all thought patterns. When a thought arises we may take note of it, but there is no need to become emotionally involved. We let go of it just as we might release the string attached to a helium-filled balloon and let the balloon drift away. Then we gently guide the mind back to the object of meditation. Gradually the mind becomes empty of all thoughts save the object of meditation. When this occurs we can experience a mental state diametrically opposed to stress—one free from worry, concern, conflict, and pressure.

The meditative state also has profound physiological effects. Mental activity always precedes and directs physiological activity: we think about doing something and then fractions of a second later we do it physically. In fact, all thoughts create a physiological response—even if we merely think about throwing a ball, there is a slight but definitely measurable response in the arm muscles. If we think about something that angers us, a subtle echo of this takes place throughout the muscles and the nervous system.

Not surprisingly, many people claim that they attain a state of total muscular relaxation when they empty the mind, and there are no thoughts and feelings dashing about on the field of consciousness. Because the mind is calm during the meditative state, there is an opportunity for relaxation of the muscles and a balancing of the nervous system. The body achieves a state of physiological quietness, and these physiological changes are far-reaching, involving muscles, blood chemistry, brain waves, breathing, the cardiovascular system, and metabolism. Thus, harmony is established at all levels of the body.

In addition, the effects of meditation tend to persist throughout the day: we retain some awareness of a peaceful state within and are able to choose to recreate aspects of that state during the day. We are no longer slaves to our own responses, but have the ability to modify our reactions. We can recall the peace of our last meditation and can look forward to the next. Thus, meditation becomes a peaceful pause in the otherwise hectic flow of life.

There are also techniques for maintaining the essence of the meditative experience in our ongoing daily lives. One of these is called "meditation in action," and it is a technique for transforming the quality of our actions in a manner that can dramatically reduce stress throughout the day. This technique will be described in greater detail below.

Let us consider the effect of meditation on the unconscious mind. This unknown portion of the mind is a significant source of stress. At the unconscious level we often have needs or mental conflicts that are too frightening, painful, or dangerous for us to deal with at a conscious level. For example, we may have fear about our adequacy, anger at someone close to us, or sadness about a rejection. These strong impressions, while too emotionally charged for us to deal with consciously, may still have subtle and powerful effects on our feelings, behavior, or interactions with others. We may find ourselves experiencing feelings or behaving in a way that we don't understand. Thus, unconscious conflict may contribute to mental unrest, strong negative emotions, or impulsive behavior, all of which can intensify the stress that we experience.

Generally, it is difficult to examine these more unconscious sources of stress. During meditation, however, we can look within and at the same time feel mentally and physically secure and comfortable. This allows some of our unconscious concerns to come into our awareness.

During meditation we may find a memory emerging about some earlier event to which we had not really paid much attention at the time, and yet now we become aware that it made a deep impression. Or, as is often true during longer periods of meditation, some powerful memory or image from months or even years in the past may emerge and the hurt or pain connected with that experience may be clearly felt.

When this occurs, we may understand how we have unknowingly carried this experience with us and become aware of the emotional charge that has accompanied it and continued to subtly influence our stress levels. Thus, meditation assists us in developing insight into our unconscious processes.

Meditation not only provides an opportunity to safely and less defensively become aware of these unconscious impressions, it also allows us to free ourselves from their influence if we can neutrally witness the impressions as they arise.

On one level, meditation is a cleansing technique for the unconscious mind. We allow unconscious impressions to come forward, we witness them, and then release them. This occurs naturally and spontaneously as we meditate. The intensity of this cleansing can vary; sometimes during meditation many impressions from the unconscious rise and are released, while at other times relatively few impressions come forward.

With a regular practice of meditation we have a daily vehicle for the continual release of unconscious conflict. In this manner we become "insiders" gently and at a comfortable pace, gaining in inner awareness and releasing unconscious material that may contribute to stress.

In the system of meditation, stress and suffering are considered to be equivalent. Suffering is avoided by stilling the mind, and this is accomplished by first relaxing the body and balancing the breath and nervous system. Then, we calm the conscious waves in the mind and finally we still the deeper currents and whirlpools in the unconscious. Thus, suffering and stress can be avoided.

But meditation is more than a method for preventing stress; during the deepest levels of meditation an aspect of ourselves emerges that is creative and health endowing. In the meditative traditions it is felt that when we still all the habitual and conditioned aspects of the mind our true essence emerges. This true self is characterized as having a natural self esteem, a sense of unity and connectedness with all around it, and a direction and purpose in life. This emergent true self has all the characteristics associated with an integrated personality and increased resistance to the stressors of daily life.

This whole idea of uncovering our potentials to increase our fitness may seem somewhat foreign, for most of us hold an additive assumption about health and hardiness. We believe that we become better, stronger, hardier, and healthier by adding things to our life. We believe that we become stronger only by acquiring training, skills, and experiences in the outer world. In this view, we must acquire things from outside in order to become full and complete.

In meditation, the model is quite different: we actually become by uncovering. Within each of us is an essence, a true self waiting to be unfolded. This self is free from conditioning, habits, and suggestion. As the conscious and unconscious thought waves are stilled, this essence is uncovered. The very nature of this essence is wholeness, integration, and freedom from suffering or stress.

In the book *Zen Mind, Beginner's Mind,* Shunryu Suzuki explains that this essence is our true nature. He writes, "When we forget ourselves, we actually are the true activity of the big existence or reality itself. When we realize this fact, there is no problem whatsoever in this world, and we can enjoy our life without feeling any difficulties. The purpose of our practice [of meditation] is to be aware of this fact."[2]

In the tradition of meditation, this inner essence is referred to as the Self. As Swami Rama writes in *Lectures on Yoga,* "The ultimate goal of meditation is to experience the Self or Atman. The Self is pure consciousness. The experience of Self is a state of transcendent knowledge and bliss. It is that state beyond time, space, and causation, which has been variously called samadhi, nirvana, cosmic consciousness and so on. When the mind is completely centered for an extended period of time, when it is not distracted by various thoughts or external objects, we become aware of the essence of our being, the Atman."[3]

There are several results of the emergence of the true nature or true Self: first of all, the more we become aware of the true Self the more our desires and aspirations are likely to change. Old habits that have contributed to stress may drop away. A preference for that which is beneficial and healthful may grow. We may spontaneously find ourselves beginning to eat better, sleep better, and exercise more easily. Simultaneously, negative and harmful thought patterns fall away because we become aware of how these habits cloud our experience of the true Self.

But more important, with the emergence of the true Self, we begin to feel within ourselves an increasingly clear sense of purpose in life. We know what we want to do and we know what is right for us. Certain goals in the areas of work, learning, and relationships emerge. It becomes easier to establish priorities and organize our time around them. We begin to partake more and more of the joy, enthusiasm, and positive emotional states that accompany our efforts to achieve our goals and objectives in life.

These positive emotions create a state of well-being and health. Striving toward our heartfelt goals also leads to a continual transformation in our personality. Seen in this context, meditation not only helps us to overcome stress but also leads to enhanced levels of health.

There are, however, other interesting effects of meditation. One of these is the manner in which meditation also affects our experience of time. Typically we experience time in a very linear fashion: one event follows the other, one day follows the last; the hours, minutes, and days follow one another inexorably. This linear view of time is intertwined with the experience of stress. We may feel "time frustration," the feeling that there is not enough time or hours in the day to accomplish the things that need to be done. Or we may feel "time pressure," the drive to squeeze more and more activities into less and less time.

Time pressure and time frustration are cardinal signs of the Type A (coronary prone) behavior pattern. This attitude toward life is associated with increased vulnerability to stress. Constant time pressure seems to lead to underlying feelings of impatience, frustration, and anger. We feel constantly vigilant in an attempt to squeeze more and more into the allotted time. Life becomes a constant struggle against time and we always feel some degree of pressure.

During meditation our experience of time changes. As we prepare for meditation, we bring our focus into the present by becoming relaxed, comfortable, and open to the here and now. Then, as we begin to focus on the chosen object of meditation, we may notice that certain time pressure thoughts begin to move into our awareness. For example, we may think of things we need to do today and tomorrow. But rather than becoming hooked by these thoughts, we let go and keep our attention focused on the present and on the object of meditation.

As the meditative state deepens, our experience of the here and now grows. In the tradition of meditation it is said that time is a construct of the mind: time is the space between two thoughts. When there is only one continuous flowing thought, then there is no experience of linear time and no time pressure. We feel mindful and complete in the present.

This "present-centeredness" may continue after meditation: meditators often find that they feel pleasantly focused in the here and now. This experience frees us of time frustration and may also enhance our performance of whatever we are doing at the moment.

Preoccupation with either the past or the future has always been seen in the meditative traditions as an enemy of excellence in the present. We miss the richness of present experience, we fail to see crucial aspects of the current situation, and we are unaware of possible options when we lack present-centeredness. In the pure meditative tradition a teacher may note the student's ability to be in the here and now as a barometer of progress. Being fully in the present and free of conflict enriches our experience and allows for the fullest expression of our potentials, allowing us to move gracefully amid the demands of time.

Present-centeredness also creates an arena for change. Change occurs in the present: whatever we feel about the past or future, real change can occur only in the present as we organize ourselves differently. When we practice meditation we create a state of quiet and present-centeredness on all levels of being. This experience changes the way our entire system organizes itself, and as we become mindful in the present, we change.

This change occurs in several ways. The first involves the principle of moving away from the negative. When we are quiet and present-centered we often obtain insight into those behaviors, thoughts, and feelings that create imbalances. Noticing these effects, we begin to move away from such harmful and stress-producing patterns. But we usually require a state of quiet to become aware of these effects.

The second principle involves moving toward the positive. In meditation we come to experience a state of peace, inner contentment, and integration. We are easily and naturally attracted toward this experience and act to repeat it. We sense something new and positive emerging and we move toward it. Again, a state of awareness and present-centeredness is the prerequisite for this process.

Typically, there is so much noise and distraction in contemporary life that only the loudest of signals are heard. Sometimes, for example, we do not notice our overall tension until we have a headache, or we do not move toward expanding our potentials until we have achieved external recognition.

Meditation creates the conditions of quiet and present-centeredness where these two mechanisms of change can become much more active and effective. The meditative state simply allows us to have greater sensitivity for and insight into those factors in our lives that are producing stress and those that are stimulating growth. With this enhanced sensitivity and insight, change occurs spontaneously.

Meditation also provides us with an experience of simplicity. As both mind and body become quiet and we become absorbed in the object of meditation, our mental processes become simplified. We do not have the background static of past worries, future anxieties, and ongoing rumination to complicate the way we see, hear, and feel things. Consequently we tend to perceive the world directly and more realistically. When we witness we see things as they are without looking at them from the perspective of our mental and perceptual habits and free of the influence of automatic emotional reactions.

This simplicity in perception, when combined with present-centeredness, allows us to be spontaneous in our behavior and free from inner conflict. We are able to respond more effectively to the reality of what is happening both inside and outside ourselves.

When we are free of conflict it is natural to respond

clearly, directly, and decisively to events around us. Whether we are helping others, arranging business priorities, or performing other actions, when the mind is quiet we see situations clearly, understand their richness of potentials, and we know what to do.

In a similar fashion, we are much more alert to our own physical and emotional needs. It is said that a true master is one who "eats when he is hungry and sleeps when he is tired." This is a definition of optimal health; to do this means having a clear perception of our needs for food or rest and then satisfying these needs directly.

Typically, our perception of events is conditioned by our mental habits and is tinged with doubt and conflict; different parts of ourselves vie to determine the dominant perception. Such inner conflict and rumination contribute to stress. When we meditate we create a quiet, safe place within where these diverse voices can come forward, be heard and acknowledged, and then let go. Free of the background of anxious mental chatter, the resulting quiet mind is focused and powerful.

Ultimately, the practice of meditation develops trust in our self-correcting and self-healing mechanisms. It is axiomatic in the great traditions of self-development that individuals have an inherent capability to grow and heal themselves. For this to occur, there are three necessary factors: we must turn our attention inward, we must attend to the present, and we must proceed at a pace that is safe and comfortable for us.

Meditation provides all three of these conditions. Because our attention is directed inward, we are aware of what we are feeling and experiencing. Because we let go of the past and future, we become increasingly present-centered. And because meditation is built on relaxation, we keep ourselves comfortable and can explore inner material as we are ready to do so. Thus, the practice of meditation gives us an ongoing process for overcoming stress and fostering personal growth.

It is also useful to compare formal meditation to meditation in action: during formal meditation we prepare carefully, assume the correct posture, shut down all other activities, and then, in a state of physical stillness, devote ourselves totally to meditation for a specific length of time.

In the practice of meditation in action, certain aspects of the meditative process are applied to our ongoing experience. Foremost among these is the concept of witnessing. During meditation we witness the thoughts, images, and memories that arise without reacting excessively. Thus we train a part of the mind to impartially watch the flow of mental events. We can use this skill during daily life; a part of our mind watches the emotions, thoughts, and impressions without reacting.

This serves as a calm center in the storm of the day's activities. It allows us a greater degree of choice in how we react to events around us. The witnessing process keeps a portion of our awareness turned inward, affording us the opportunity to adjust our responses at any time.

A more structured type of meditation in action involves actually focusing on some object of meditation while we are active. For example, we may repeat our mantra inwardly or focus on and count the breaths. Our first impression might be that this practice would be distracting and disruptive, but, in fact, as we use it, the effect is grounding and centering. It brings us into the present, creates a mental calmness, and allows us to be more mindful as we act.

In summary, there are many reasons why meditation can be considered the quintessential technique for overcoming stress and transforming the self: it calms the mind, transforms perception, releases inner conflict, and enhances our awareness of what is helpful or harmful to us.

When meditation becomes a regular part of our life we have begun a gradual, cumulative process that creates a nourishing quiet for body and mind—the best antidote to stress. Simultaneously, meditation promotes an unfolding of our truest nature and most dynamic potentials.

SECTION II.

A New Understanding of Stress

CHAPTER 8

The Practice of Meditation

John R. Harvey, Ph.D.

Meditation is the calm, unbroken, one-pointed flow of concentration upon a subtle inner focus. Regular, systematic practice of a time-tested method of meditation is necessary to actually attain a true meditative state. There are a number of practical guidelines and preparatory steps that are quite helpful in establishing the effective practice of meditation. The following instructions may, at first, seem rather detailed and lengthy, but in a short time they can become familiar and flow into a smooth progression of steps that systematically leads to a meditative state. First of all, it is important to choose a setting that is conducive to meditation. A quiet part of your home where you will not be disturbed is ideal. This spot should be well ventilated and the temperature should be comfortable. It is also beneficial if the setting is attractive and appealing.

Another important consideration is to set aside a definite time for the practice of meditation. Early morning, at sunset, and in the evening before going to bed are generally considered the best times for meditation. Select one or two times when you can regularly meditate and stay with these times. When you do this your mind and body will spontaneously prepare for meditation and you will begin to form a positive habit. Select a time when other responsibilities will not interfere with your meditation. Regularity in practice is very important, as the effects of meditation are cumulative. Even if unexpected events crowd your schedule, you are better off meditating for at least a few minutes at your regular time than missing a session.

Traditionally, in the East, meditation was seen as a very important action and the notion of preparation included physical cleanliness. In fact, you will feel fresher and more relaxed if you take a shower or bath or wash your face and hands before sitting for meditation. Meditation is easiest when your body is not preoccupied with digesting food, so it is advisable to meditate before eating or at least several hours after a major meal.

Dress in loose comfortable clothing. Remove or loosen any items of apparel that restrict your body or create pressure. Remove glasses and hard contact lenses and take off your shoes. During the quiet of meditation, your body's metabolism tends to slow down so you may want to place a shawl over your shoulders for warmth.

You will be able to sit more comfortably for meditation if you precede your practice with some gentle exercises. Also, your feet and legs will be less likely to fall asleep if you stimulate them with some light exercise before sitting. A brief relaxation in the corpse pose (see Chapter 2) will further assist you in releasing any tension from the muscles and in preparing your body to be still and comfortable during meditation.

The next step is to select a meditation posture that is right for you. The posture should allow you to sit in a straight, comfortable, and steady manner. One option is to sit on the edge of a straight-backed chair. In this position, let your knees be shoulder-width apart, your heels underneath the knees, your hands resting on your knees or thighs, and your thighs parallel to the floor. This is the friendship pose (see figure 1).

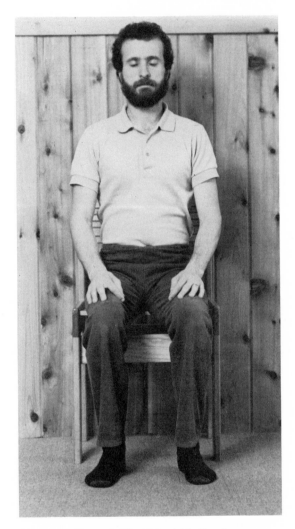

Figure 1 (The Friendship Pose)

Friendship Pose:

Sit on a straight-backed chair, keeping the head, neck, and trunk straight and placing the hands on the knees. The legs should not be crossed and the feet should be firmly placed on the ground.

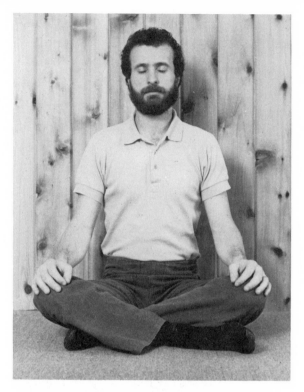

Figure 2 (The Easy Pose)

The Easy Pose:

Sitting with the head, neck, and trunk straight, place the left foot beneath the right knee and the right foot beneath the left knee. Each knee rests on the opposite foot. Place the hands on the corresponding knees.

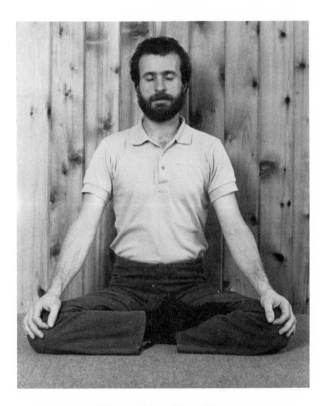

Figure 3 (Auspicious Pose)

The Auspicious Pose:

This posture is similar to the easy pose except that the legs are positioned differently to provide an even firmer and steadier base. While seated on the floor, bend the left leg at the knee and place the sole of the left foot against the right thigh. Place the right foot on top of the left calf, and put the outer edge of the right foot and the toes between the left thigh and calf muscles. Only the right big toe should be visible. Pull the toes of the left foot up between the right thigh and calf so that the left big toe is visible. Place the hands on the corresponding knees and straighten the head, neck, and trunk.

You can also sit on the floor in a cross-legged position such as the easy pose or the auspicious pose. The easy pose is particularly useful for beginners, older people, or individuals who are not particularly limber, while the auspicious pose is somewhat more physically challenging. (See figures 2 and 3.) For either of these poses, you may find it quite helpful to wedge a firm pillow or folded blanket under the buttocks to support the lower back and make the posture more comfortable.

Once you have selected a meditation posture, use it consistently so that your body can become accustomed to that position and with practice you can perfect it. Each time you sit for meditation make sure that your head, neck, and trunk are properly aligned. Gently close your eyes so that you are not distracted by external sights. Relax and settle comfortably into the pose, sitting tall and centered.

Then you can use certain breathing techniques to balance the nervous system and bring the mind to a calm, alert state conducive to meditation. Begin by establishing even, smooth diaphragmatic breathing. As you exhale, gently bring your abdomen inward; as you inhale, allow your abdomen to move outward. Be aware of any shallowness, jerkiness, pauses, or noise in your breath. Allow your breathing to be deep and slow and within your comfortable capacity. Allow your breathing to flow smoothly and without interruption or hesitation between inhalations and exhalations. Find a regular rate and rhythm for your breath and let the exhalation and inhalation become equal in length.

After learning to establish even, diaphragmatic breathing, there are other breathing techniques that you can use to further refine the mental state. Among these are the Complete Breath and Alternate Nostril Breathing. The Complete Breath is a simple cleansing technique designed to remove excessive carbon dioxide and bring in adequate oxygen. It leaves one feeling refreshed and energized.

Alternate Nostril Breathing is particularly effective in refining the mental state and producing a state of balance and calmness that greatly facilitates meditation. Directions for practicing these two techniques are given at the end of Chapter 4. Anywhere from three to ten complete breaths and one to three rounds of Alternate Nostril Breathing are good preparation for meditation.

Once you have made the breath even and calm, the next step is to draw your awareness inward and let go of external preoccupations. Again, relax any muscular tension and keep your body as quiet as possible for the duration of the practice. Survey your body systematically from the top of your head to your toes, releasing any tension or discomfort that you might observe along the way. Then, very slowly bring your awareness back from your toes to the top of your head.

Begin the practice of breath awareness: feel your breath as it flows through the nostrils—warm and moist as you exhale, cool and dry as you inhale. You may notice that the air is flowing slightly more freely through one nostril and less freely through the other. Observe the flow of your breath through the more open, active nostril for several breaths. Next, observe the flow of your breath through the less open, passive nostril for several breaths. Then bring your awareness to the point where your upper lip meets the area between the nostrils and continue to observe the flow of the breath. As you maintain your attention you are practicing breath awareness meditation, which can be used to great benefit, helping you to develop awareness of a calm center within.

After you have practiced breath awareness meditation for a period of time you may develop an interest in obtaining an even more profound experience of inner peace and quiet. A natural progression at this point is to begin the practice of mantra meditation. A mantra is a subtle sound vibration that helps develop a deeper state of meditation. Usually a personal mantra that is suitable for an individual is given by a qualified meditation teacher. However, there is a universal mantra that can be used by all beginning meditators. This mantra is "Soham" and it means, "I am that" or "I am that true or real self." This mantra is useful in helping the student to understand and unfold his true nature. To practice this mantra, mentally hear the sound "so" as you inhale and "ham" (pronounced hum) as you exhale. Silently observe the mantra as it flows with the breathing. Relax your body, breath and mind in the mantra. Let yourself become absorbed in the mantra awareness, maintaining focus only on the inner sound, Soham.

As you meditate, avoid identifying with the thought forms that come into the mind. Be an objective witness to them. Remain established in the mantra. Simply allow memories, images, and feelings to flow by without reacting. Don't analyze, critique, or be swayed by the contents of the mind. Remain focused on the mantra. If your attention should drift away, avoid overreacting or judging yourself. Simply return your focus gently to the mantra. Stay with the mantra. Keep bringing the mind back to the mantra when it wanders. Ultimately, meditation is quite simple: one becomes absorbed in the mantra, the object of meditation.

One should practice meditation for as long as is comfortable, beginning with five to ten minutes and working up to twenty or thirty minutes. The key is to practice gently, within your capacity and extend the time in a gradual and easy manner. Beginning meditators are often concerned with keeping track of the time so they know when to end their meditation. Ideally, you can trust your own internal clock to let you know when ten or twenty minutes have elapsed.

When you have finished, slowly bring your palms up to cover your eyes. Open your eyes into your palms, and gradually bring your hands away, returning your attention to the external world. You may want to stretch your limbs as you get up from your meditation posture. When you resume your activities, work toward maintaining an awareness of the breath and mantra throughout the day. Maintaining a calm center within while acting effectively in daily life is called "meditation in action." The breath and mantra can be the core of this calm center.

Once mastered, the practice of meditation is very effective in reducing stress. Through daily practice, the nervous system is calmed; emotional control and self-understanding are increased. Feelings of anxiety and tension are reduced, and the self-talks that produce these states become less influential. The mantra is a positive and uplifting thought form that brings you to an awareness of peace within and at the same time introduces you to deeper levels of your being. Mantra meditation helps you to uncover your latent potentials. It also initiates a process of increasing inner awareness that assists in formulating a perspective on life based on your inner experience. You can then begin to enjoy a greater sense of meaning and purpose in life. Thus, meditation, which at first is practiced as a stress reduction technique, becomes a vehicle for personal transformation. Feelings of frustration, isolation, and alienation decrease and a sense of peace, contentment, and inner balance grows.

CHAPTER 9
Stress: A New Perspective

Phil Nuernberger, Ph.D.

Stress is now considered to be the major causal factor of physical and mental disease, behavioral dysfunctions, and social problems. Our understanding of just what is meant by the term "stress," however, has not kept pace with the recognition of its importance. Modern theories on stress are incomplete and often incompatible with each other. Each tends to focus on only one aspect of stress, without maintaining an overall perspective of the different aspects of human functioning. These theories fail to provide a logical and consistent framework of human functioning from which human dysfunctions such as stress can be logically and successfully explained and understood.

The predominant and most familiar model of stress is found in the General Adaptation Syndrome (GAS) theory of Hans Selye.[1,2] Selye first defines "stress" as "the nonspecific response of the body to any demand made upon it." A central mediating factor is the intensity of the demand and the consequent physiological response (which Selye calls stress) to this intensity. Selye then refers to any positive outcome of this response as "Eustress." When the body's response has negative consequences, (for example, leading to a disruptive or pathological condition) it is referred to as "Distress." Thus, according to Selye, "stress" is an unavoidable condition referring to the body's physiological response to any demand.

More particularly, the General Adaptation Syndrome (GAS) conceptualizes the stress response as existing in three stages. The first, the Alarm stage, is the activation of the arousal response as the individual reacts to a perceived threat. This entails the so-called "fight or flight" response, and is predominantly seen as the arousal response that prepares the body for action. This response is regulated by the sympathetic nervous system, which is the part of the autonomic nervous system that mediates arousal in the body.

The second stage is called Adaptation and consists of the body's compensatory response to fight or flight arousal. It is, in general, the body's attempt to return to homeostasis.

If the Alarm reaction is continually activated due to unresolved or continuous threat (worries, concerns or fears), the body's resources are depleted. This brings on Fatigue, the third stage of the GAS. This state can evolve into a dangerous depletion of bodily resources, resulting in breakdown, disease, and even death of the organism. Thus, Selye defines "Distress" as the physiological response of sustained sympathetic dominance in which the body's resources are depleted, resulting in pathology, disease, and even death.

Similar to Selye's position is the psychophysiological theory that "stress" is that which stimulates the physiological systems, causing the physical symptoms of stress disorders. Both Selye's and the psychophysiological theory depend primarily on the impact of sustained or intense arousal to define stress.

There are several major limitations to the GAS framework that have led to a number of logical problems, and prevent us from achieving a more sophisticated understanding of stress. First of all, the GAS is based primarily on sympathetic arousal and does not deal adequately with the less dramatic but equally powerful role and influence of parasympathetic functioning. This is also true of the psychophysiological theory of stress. The GAS stages of Alarm, Adaptation and Fatigue are described almost exclusively in terms of arousal, over-utilization, and depletion of bodily resources. This equation of stress with arousal (sympathetic dominance) ignores the harmful effects of extreme parasympathetic dominance. Consequently, neither theory can account for such stress conditions as depression, passivity, or withdrawal. For example, depression does not lead to a depletion of bodily resources, but rather to a failure to utilize these resources. This is an entirely different kind of dysfunction in which the end result could be, and often is, as fatal as the end result of fatigue.

The equation of stress with arousal has led to the logical absurdity of "good stress" and "bad stress," which is the source of much confusion. For example, we often hear that a certain amount of stress is not only useful but necessary for maintaining motivation and performance. Yet we know that stress can be very harmful, leading to such conditions as coronary vascular disease. On one hand, stress is good because the consequences are good, for example, we feel good, get more work done. On the other hand, stress is bad when the consequences are harmful, that is, heart attack, headaches, or divorce. The difference between good and bad is determined only by the consequences. This provides no predictive power whatsoever, and is essentially useless as a scientific theory or as a practical guide. If you are unable to tell the difference between "good stress" and "bad stress" until after the heart attack, the difference is of no value to you, or to the scientist, doctor, or researcher. Simply adding new terms, such as "Eustress" and "Distress," only adds to the confusion and does little to clarify the issue.

Secondly, the GAS model, based solely on physiological response patterning, ignores the determinant role of mental functioning. The autonomic and other physiological responses studied by Selye are regulated primarily by limbic functioning. The limbic system is subject to control and influence by the higher cortical processes, that is, the thinking process. In short, as Roger Sperry succinctly states, mental events control physical events.[3] The GAS model treats autonomic processes as if they really were autonomous, which was the assumption at the time Selye formulated his theory. In contrast, there are two minor theories, the psychodynamic and cognitive theories, that do focus on mental activity as the determining source of stress. However, as Barbara Brown points out, they fail to define and explain the intervening variables between the mental event and the physiological response.[4]

A third limitation inherent in the GAS model and other theories of stress is a dependency upon a mechanistic application of homeostasis. Homeostasis was a central concept in Walter B. Cannon's original work on stress, and it still retains the flavor of a constancy mechanism. Homeostasis, as generally used, is a concept that applies to a closed system, such as a machine. Current theories on stress generally treat human functioning as if it were mechanistic, that is, a closed system. Cannon's definition of homeostasis as "the coordinated physiological processes which maintain most of the steady states in the organism" is an accurate description of a closed system. Human beings are more accurately described by systems theory as an "open system," a system that is in constant interaction with its environment, being modified by and in turn modifying that environment. A mechanistic "closed system" description fails to take into account the "dynamic equilibrium" characteristic of human functioning. The principles of open system,[5] such as *equifinality* (the reaching of a goal through a variety of initial conditions and ways), *harmonization* (an integrated balancing) of energy and processes, and the ability to perform (obtain) work in states of complete harmonization or dynamic equilibrium, all more accurately describe human functioning. Furthermore, an open systems approach is of necessity holistic, involving all aspects of human functioning, and all planes. Current conceptualizations of stress either treat the individual (or the physiological response) as a passive recipient of demands or influences from the environment (internal or external), or fail to explain the dynamic principles involved in the mind/body interaction. These models of stress are much too narrowly based, leading to conflict and confusion in terms and concepts, thus limiting their usefulness and power as explanatory frameworks.

What is needed is a comprehensive (holistic) framework that accounts for the various aspects and levels of human functioning, and that can provide the practical elements of prediction and control. One such framework has its basis in the comprehensive analysis of human functioning found in yoga and Vedantic psychological sciences. Widely misunderstood in the Western world, yoga is a highly experimental and empirical science that demands the utmost discrimination and verification. Its discerning analysis and understanding of human functioning underlie the seemingly remarkable controls over mental and physical events and the superordinary abilities demonstrated by yoga masters.[6] It is within this comprehensive framework that stress—human dysfunctioning—can be more completely understood.

Any framework will to some extent be a simplification, but it should have the advantage of illustrating the principles that govern human functioning. The model should also clarify the complex interactive processes of consciousness, mind, and matter (body), as well as their interaction with the environment. Briefly, the model is as follows: we are concerned with three interpenetrating levels, called *koshas* or sheaths, the physical sheath, the energy sheath, and the mental sheath. The first and most obvious sheath or level is the physical body, including those physiological response systems regulated primarily by the autonomic nervous system (ANS). The ANS and the response systems are influenced by many things, such as glandular function, physical activity, and diet. The autonomic system, however, is itself controlled by the central nervous system, and in particular the limbic system. The limbic system, is, in turn, influenced by a variety of events, including autonomic and sensory motor functioning. However, it is the higher cortical functions in the cerebral cortex, the "thinking processes" that directly mediate what occurs in the limbic system.

The second level is the subtle substructure of energy. This energy is the underlying reality of the physical body. From physics we know that what appears to our senses as a solid object is in reality not solid at all, but a complex patterning of atomic and sub-atomic energy structures. Our body is no different than any other object. This level of human functioning is called the *pranic* sheath. The term "prana" means literally the "first unit of energy," or the most subtle form of energy.

Western science and medicine have little knowledge of the dynamics of this level of functioning, and still treat the body as if the biochemical level was the ultimate level. Curiously enough, even the physicist somehow forgets the underlying energy reality when dealing with his own body. This pranic level, however, has been the focus of intense study in yoga science, as well as other Oriental sciences. The pranic sheath is seen as the link between body and mind, and functions within predictable and systematic parameters. The major vehicle of prana is the breath which, as we shall see later, plays a significant role in the regulation of both autonomic and central nervous system functioning.

The third level is that of mental functioning, and is referred to as the mental sheath. For our present purposes, we are defining only one level as the mental sheath. In later development and discussion two more levels will be defined that detail more subtle aspects of human functioning. It is on the level of this third sheath that sensory input is organized and given meaning, mentation occurs, and memory and emotions have their play. The mind is understood as a distinct and separate reality from the body, with extension into time and space, and is not to be confused with mere neurological activity. Through the direction and regulation of energy, whether on the subtle plane or on the gross physical plane, the mind regulates and absolutely controls all physiological processes.[7]

There is reciprocal influence occurring at all times both between levels and within levels. The process functions as an *interpenetrating hierarchical structure,* that has its most apparent parameters in the physical sheath and becomes increasingly more subtle as one moves toward mind. On the physical plane, for example, regulatory control is hierarchically structured so that each level controls that which is lower, and in turn influences the level(s) superior to it. Thus, we see that the autonomic system is regulated by the limbic system, which in turn is regulated by the higher cortical processes. Yet within any one level, each particular system has some capacity for self-regulation.

Between systems, the more subtle level is the controlling agent. For example, the pranic sheath sustains the physical sheath, and the mental sheath sustains the pranic sheath. This can best be understood as interpenetration. Figure 1 illustrates this principle. The three sheaths are pictured as concentric rings—the outer ring is the physical sheath, the second ring is the *pranic* sheath, and the third, innermost ring, is the mental sheath. As the illustration shows, the mental sheath permeates both the pranic sheath

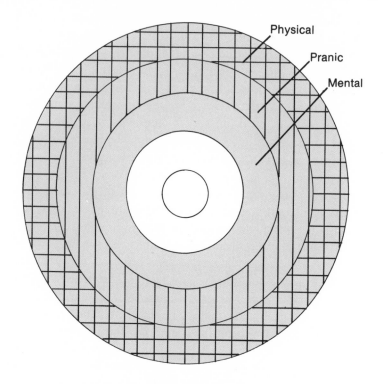

Figure 1
Three Interpenetrating Levels of Functioning or Sheaths as Presented in Yoga Science.

and the physical sheath. This interpenetration allows for both absolute control by higher sheaths and communication between the sheaths. Figure 1 also points out the role of energy as the defining interactional agent between mind and body.

One further principle is the necessity of harmonization of physical, mental, and energy processes in a dynamic balance to allow the human to function at a high level without creating problems. Disharmonization implies dysfunction. Harmonization occurs in a variety of ways and utilizes a variety of systems or conditions, and it is best defined by the principle of equifinality. The mental activities that establish inner harmonious habit formation are awareness, and will (the capacity to consciously direct energy to achieve a certain end).

Given this brief overview we will now examine the causes and effects of stress on each level. Since the autonomic system regulates our internal environment, it is this system that determines the physiological parameters of the stress response. This system is called autonomic because it can function without conscious direction or awareness. However, that does not mean that it operates independently of the central nervous system and mental activity.

The autonomic system is comprised of two anatomically distinct nervous systems, the sympathetic and parasympathetic. The sympathetic system mediates the inner physiological mechanisms of arousal and is associated with outward activity involving muscular exertion and large expenditures of energy. Its emergency function is life-protective, and it has the capacity to function on a moment's notice, emitting a sudden, large, and coordinated discharge through its extensive interconnections of all the nerve fibers in the ganglia along the spinal column.

The parasympathetic system regulates the housekeeping work of the body—the inward activities of nourishment and excretion, the repair of tissues, and the build-up of energy and fuel supplies for the next period of outward action. It is organized along a more site-specific basis without the overall instantaneous capacity of the sympathetic system.

The organs and organ systems are, by and large, innervated by both sympathetic and parasympathetic systems, and this is referred to as reciprocal innervation. Although anatomically distinct, the two systems are continuously engaged in a balancing act that indicates a very high level of mutual influence and communication. At the autonomic level, this probably occurs as a result of the reciprocal innervation but, more importantly, occurs in the nerve plexuses. These plexuses are groupings of nerve fibers from each system and are found along the vertical axis of the body, from the base of the spine to the head, in front of the vertebral column. Although the nerves from the two systems do not interconnect, we can expect a high degree of mutual influence and interaction to take place through the electrical or energy fields that they create. This would seem to be an extremely important part of the energy and communication systems that occur on subtle levels throughout the body. In healthy functioning, these two systems work to harmonize physiological activity to meet the demands made upon the body. Understanding this natural capacity for harmonization or dynamic balance is necessary for a comprehensive and functional understanding of stress.

As discussed above, stress is typically and mistakenly identified with arousal. It is well established that sustained or intense sympathetic dominance is very stressful and can lead to exhaustion, pathology, and even death. However, sustained or intense parasympathetic dominance also leads to pathology and death. For example, certain illnesses, such as asthma and duodenal ulcers, are directly associated with abnormal parasympathetic activity. Both asthma and duodenal ulcers involve changes associated with increased vagus nerve activity, which is the major parasympathetic nerve. There are two distinct autonomic responses to discomfort or perceived threat in the environment. Increased arousal is one response, adequately described as the "fight or flight" response and the three stages of the GAS. Another response to discomfort is increased parasympathetic dominance, either as an organ-specific manifestation or as a generalized response resulting in syndromes such as depression. A third, most common response is a mixed or combined response, consisting of inappropriate overall arousal and inappropriate inhibition in a specific organ system.

If we recognize that there can be a pathological over-dominance of parasympathetic activity, then we must re-formulate our concept of stress. There are a significant number of individuals who respond to threat with passive withdrawal, or what may be called the "possum response." That is, instead of preparing to fight or run away when faced with a threatening situation, they just roll over and play dead. Their response to fear is not arousal, but inhibition. This is marked by the typical characteristics of extreme parasympathetic discharge—decreased physiolog-ical functioning, loss of skeletal tone, mental lassitude, inactivity, and eventual depression.

The possum response may be originally rooted in the failure of autonomic arousal to adequately cope with what was perceived as environmental threats or demands, and it may have developed as a counter-attempt to control them. For example, there is Seligman's work with "learned help-lessness," and the consequent pathology and even death that resulted from this learning.[8] The possum response may also be a learned response developed from a sociali-zation process in which social dominance/submission is-sues were important determinants. More likely, the pos-sum response is a complex syndrome involving not only constitutional predisposition and organ-specific weak-nesses, but also subtle psychological and learning factors. In any event, it is evident that a significant number of people react to a threat with a response that can be explained only as parasympathetic dominance.

There appear to be consistent stages that characterize parasympathetic dominance that are similar to the stages defined by the GAS theory involving arousal. Table 1 below presents a summary of the stages of both sympa-thetic and parasympathetic reactivity.

The first stage, the Alarm stage, is characterized by the

Table 1
Stages of Stress Reaction Involving Both Sympathetic and Parasympathetic Dominance

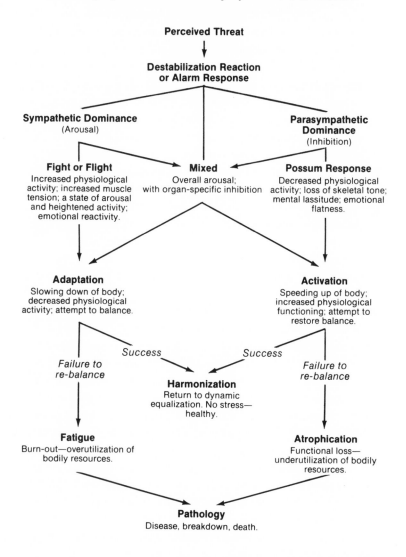

Perceived Threat

Destabilization Reaction or Alarm Response

Sympathetic Dominance
(Arousal)

Parasympathetic Dominance
(Inhibition)

Fight or Flight
Increased physiological activity; increased muscle tension; a state of arousal and heightened activity; emotional reactivity.

Mixed
Overall arousal; with organ-specific inhibition

Possum Response
Decreased physiological activity; loss of skeletal tone; mental lassitude; emotional flatness.

Adaptation
Slowing down of body; decreased physiological activity; attempt to balance.

Activation
Speeding up of body; increased physiological functioning; attempt to restore balance.

Failure to re-balance

Success

Success

Failure to re-balance

Harmonization
Return to dynamic equalization. No stress—healthy.

Fatigue
Burn-out—overutilization of bodily resources.

Atrophication
Functional loss—underutilization of bodily resources.

Pathology
Disease, breakdown, death.

possum response. The second stage is a process of adaptation that is characterized by increased activity that is needed to balance the inhibition. The third stage is characterized by increasing loss of functional capacity. This is not a depletion of resources as is found in the Fatigue stage of the GAS theory, but rather an atrophy of the organ capacity. This can be understood as a process similar to that occurring when muscles are no longer used or have been immobilized for a period of time. An example of the effects of this functional loss is found in the work of LeShan on the failure of immune systems in those who have suffered the loss of a loved one.[9] The high rate of pathology and even death is directly attributable to the failure of immune functioning because of the emotional trauma and subsequent inhibition (experienced as depression).

Table 1, involving both sides of the autonomic system, gives us a more comprehensive and more functionally useful definition of the physiological response parameters of stress. We may then define stress as

a state of autonomic imbalance, characterized by unrelieved or excessive dominance of either arousal or inhibition, or a complex interaction of the two. This imbalance leads to impaired (damaged) or diminished physiological and/or mental functioning.

Prolonged stress is a consistent pattern of imbalance resulting from the habitual dominance of sympathetic (fight or flight) activity or parasympathetic (possum response) activity. This pattern occurs either in particular, organ specific sites or as a generalized response pattern. In other words, stress occurs when we are out of balance. This principle is illustrated in figure 2. If we use the letter A (for autonomic) as a balance point, it becomes easy to understand the principle involved.

Healthy, nonstressful functioning is represented by a balance between sympathetic and parasympathetic activity. This balance is really a harmonization of function and

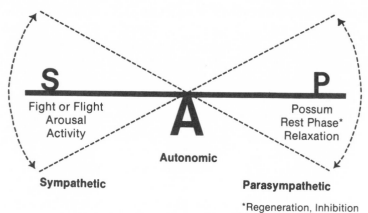

Figure 2
Balance and the Autonomic Nervous System
Source: Nuernberger: *Freedom from Stress: A Holistic Approach*

energy. The balance can be dynamic, constantly shifting from the dominance of one system to the other as required to satisfy the demands made upon the body. As long as this shifting remains fluid or dynamic, the possibility of stress is minimal. Consequently, we can have periods of arousal (or patterns of activity) that are healthy and nonstressful as long as they are balanced by periods of relaxation and rest. A state of relaxation (parasympathetic dominance), if it is not balanced by activity, can also become dysfunctional, resulting in lethargy and depression.

Balance may also take the form of complete harmonization or dynamic equilibrium between the two systems. A balanced dynamic state is created and maintained in which there is no stress, although a great deal of physical and mental activity can be accomplished during this period. An example is the resting heartbeat, which is in perfect autonomic balance and yet still pumping blood and accomplishing its job. A more complex example of this harmonization is a meditative state of mind in which the mind is alert, but the body is very relaxed.

If we understand stress to be a state of autonomic imbalance, then we can eliminate the confusion between "good" stress and "bad" stress (which is really a confusion created by equating arousal and stress). The fact that we have either arousal or inhibition does not, in and of itself, mean that we have stress. The key element in defining the physiological parameters of stress can be whether or not there exists a balance, either dynamically or as total harmonization, between sympathetic and parasympathetic activity. Stress can be operationally defined as autonomic imbalance.

Although figure 2 is helpful in illustrating the principle of balance, it is a mechanistic oversimplification of an extremely complex system of energy. It is not one or the other part of the autonomic system, as the diagram would seem to indicate, but rather an interactive process involving both. The fact that the sympathetic response is instantaneous and global, while parasympathetic activity is site-specific, allows for a complex interaction between the two at all times. Most of what we normally call disease is the result of this complex interaction between the sympathetic and parasympathetic systems. Stress, or autonomic imbalance, is also an interactive process involving both systems.

Rather than the mechanistic balance depicted in figure 2, a more fitting analogy is that of a crystal sphere representing the entire arena of autonomic functioning. The internal sphere is serviced by both the sympathetic and parasympathetic systems. In figure 3 below, when the system is in harmony (a), and there is no stress, the crystal areas are clear. When a disharmony or imbalance occurs somewhere in the system (b), for whatever reason, we have a state of stress, represented by a shading somewhere in this autonomic area. If we have prolonged or intense parasympathetic imbalance, then we may develop a disease associated with that imbalance, such as asthma or depression. If we have prolonged or intense sympathetic imbalance, we may develop a disease associated with that imbalance, such as hypertension. But always there is the interaction of sympathetic energy and parasympathetic energy or tone. As the sphere is a whole, so is our body, and we cannot divide ourselves into mechanistic pieces that operate independently from the other parts of the whole.

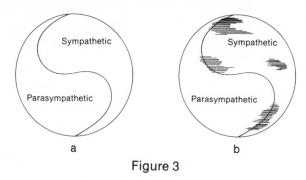

Figure 3

There are probably specific optimum balance points or even a generalized one for organs and systems involving many organs. Our organs and systems are also interconnected: if an imbalance occurs within one organ, it will affect the entire system, as well as other systems with which the initial system interacts. Conversely, if the overall autonomic response is balanced, individual subsystems will begin to achieve balance. Once we understand the principle of balance, or rather, harmonization, the problem then becomes one of understanding those events, processes, and mechanisms that lead to balance. Surprisingly, there appear to be very definite ways by which one can consciously learn to moderate and control autonomic functioning, and begin to control stress.

Energy and Breath

The concept of balance and the opportunities for stress management can be clearly seen if we examine the subtle energy structure, or second level of human functioning underlying the physical body. This energy sheath, known as the pranamaya kosha, as indicated earlier, is the interpenetrating substructure or basis for the physical level. Alterations and changes within this subtle energy structure lead to changes in the more gross physical body. According to yoga science, the major vehicle for prana (energy) is the breath, which is considered to be the "flywheel" mechanism of the body.[10,12] If the breath is disrupted (unbalanced), it will lead to disruption (imbalance) in the energy system and, thus, in the physical body. Consequently, in yoga there is a significant emphasis on proper regulation of the breath. In light of the central role of breath in the energy sheath, or pranamaya kosha, we would expect that the breathing process would play a significant role in the regulation of physiological processes. While this yogic emphasis on breathing may seem novel to the Western scientist, there is evidence to suggest that the breath does play a major regulatory role in autonomic functioning, and, thus, is a major factor in the regulation of stress, or autonomic imbalance.

Figure 4, on the following page, illustrates the balancing aspect of the autonomic nervous system. The letter A, for autonomic, is used as the balance point.

On one side is the sympathetic system regulating arousal and characterized by the alarm mechanism of "fight or flight." The parasympathetic system, regulating inhibition (rest phase), is on the other side and is characterized by the alarm mechanism of the "possum response." By understanding physiological stress as imbalance, we can reformulate the approach to the problem of stress so as to lead to a new understanding of the mind/body relationship, and to some unexpected but very powerful tools for self-regulation and control.

Until recently, Western science has given little credence to the possibility for conscious regulation of autonomic functioning. However, the yoga tradition has always

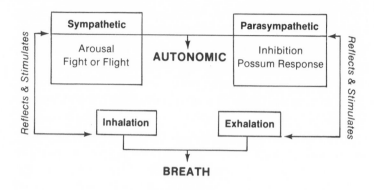

Figure 4
Breath and Autonomic Balance
Source: Nuernberger: *Freedom from Stress: A Holistic Approach*

recognized that autonomic function can be directly regulated by the mind through control of breath. As shown in figure 4, inhalation both reflects and stimulates sympathetic discharge, while exhalation reflects and stimulates parasympathetic discharge. That is, there is a subtle but direct relationship between autonomic activity and the breathing process. Consequently, autonomic tone can be directly and consciously regulated through conscious regulation of the breathing process. If the breath is disturbed, then autonomic balance is disturbed, and there is a condition of stress. Through knowledge and proper training of the breathing process, a person gains the skill to consciously and directly regulate autonomic functioning. This skill is a critical and necessary step in the self-regulation of stress.

The evidence for this relationship between the autonomic system and the breath is extensive. There are a number of studies that show that changes in respiratory patterns accompany changes in a wide variety of emotional states and mental and physical activities.[13-21]

Furthermore, specific changes in breathing patterns have been utilized in a variety of therapeutic modalities, such as bioenergetics and Gestalt therapy, and for a variety of problems, ranging from stress and anxiety management to post-surgical care and treatment of stuttering.[22-26]

There is an emerging awareness of the relationship of breathing to cardiovascular functioning. It now appears that breathing can critically influence cardiovascular functioning in several ways. Probably the most important relationship is that between breathing patterns and the electrical activity of the heart. Autonomic tone regulates the subtle exchange of potassium and sodium ions in the pacemaker cells of the heart's sino-atrial node. This exchange is what causes the heart to beat. The influence of respiratory motion on the regulation of autonomic tone can directly influence the electrical activity of the heart.[27] This influence can be so important that one researcher states that an individual who suffers a heart attack due to arrythmias can really be said to have more of a breathing problem than a heart problem.[28] An example of a pathological effect of breathing on heart functioning is the pattern of apnea found in heart patients.[29]

DasGupta, a cardiologist from the University of Chicago, points out that breathing also influences blood pressure in at least three ways.[30] Movement of the diaphragm and lungs mechanically influences the amount of blood that enters the heart. This directly affects the amount of force needed to pump blood out of the heart and is one factor in determining blood pressure. The manner of breathing also determines the blood levels of oxygen and carbon dioxide. The level of carbon dioxide affects the acid-base balance of the blood and may influence the reactivity of the blood vessels that, in turn, can affect blood pressure. A third effect on blood pressure is the effect of breathing on establishing sympathetic arousal. Chest breathing creates a state of arousal and causes sympathetic action that constricts peripheral blood vessels. This can lead directly to an elevation of blood pressure. In fact, it is chest or thoracic breathing that adversely affects our cardiovascular health.

While researchers and clinicians are increasingly aware of the relationship of the breath to various emotional, mental, and physical states, the specifics of this relationship are as yet unknown. The specific relationship of inhalation to sympathetic tone and exhalation to parasympathetic tone, so carefully studied in yoga science, is not known in Western medicine. Traditionally, yoga science has said that respiratory motion plays a major role in regulating autonomic tone, and this regulation occurs through the mechanism of the variable stimulation of the right vagus nerve. Respiratory motion, or rhythm, is regulated by a variety of factors. One of these factors is the stretch receptors located in the visceral pleura, the bronchi, bronchioles, and the alveoli. These stretch receptors transmit impulses through the vagus nerve and can both alter and maintain respiratory motion. This mechanism is known as the Hering-Breuer reflex[31] and may well be another major factor by which autonomic tone is regulated.

There is great variability in the pattern of respiratory motion. For instance, inhalation may be predominantly diaphragmatic, thoracic, or clavicular. The two major respiratory patterns, thoracic (chest breathing) and diaphragmatic, are remarkably different in their effect on both autonomic tone and ventilation perfusion efficiency. It is commonly thought that thoracic motion, or chest breathing, is associated with sympathetic arousal. Extreme examples are the pathological breathing patterns associated with hyperventilation and anxiety states.

Another major variable of respiratory motion is respiratory rate, and this, under normal circumstances, is directly related to oxygen consumption. The respiratory rate is far lower for predominantly diaphragmatic breathing than for thoracic-dominated breathing. This is because diaphragmatic breathing is a much more efficient mechanism, providing a greater efficiency of ventilation perfusion with far less muscular effort than required by thoracic-dominated patterns.[32]

Further research is needed to explain the various pathways by which the relationship between inhalation and sympathetic discharge and between exhalation and parasympathetic discharge occurs. Doubtless, the influences and interconnections are extremely complex and will require detailed examination and research.

The application of proper breathing practices is a very powerful tool in the self-regulation of stress and in the alteration of symptoms associated with stress. In yoga science, there are a variety of breathing exercises that lead to increased control over the respiratory movement. Pranayama, the conscious control of prana (energy), is achieved primarily through the conscious study and regulation of the breathing process. It should be emphasized and remembered, however, that the breath is only the major vehicle for prana, and should not be confused with the energy itself. Direct, conscious, and willful control of prana itself requires a subtlety of perception that demands a significant degree of concentration and awareness. The first step is the conscious awareness and regulation of the breathing process.

As indicated in Chapter 4, there are a number of breathing exercises that are directly applicable to the regulation of autonomic balance.[33] The most useful exercises are diaphragmatic breathing, even breathing, 2:1 breathing, alternate nostril breathing, and breath awareness. Each of these leads to enhanced control of respiratory movement and increased vital capacity.

To review briefly, the first and most essential step in effective stress management is to reestablish diaphragmatic breathing as the dominant moment-to-moment resting breathing pattern. Diaphragmatic breathing provides the most efficient ventilation perfusion and facilitates a balanced autonomic tone. Thoracic-dominated breathing leads to increased sympathetic tone and subsequent imbalance, as well as decreased ventilation perfusion efficiency and increased muscular effort. Using the diaphragm also provides a degree of control over respiratory motion that is not available through the thoracic mechanism.

Further control over respiratory movement and autonomic balance is acquired by the practice of even breathing and alternate nostril breathing. Even breathing is characterized by a steady flow of breath in which the rate of flow remains steady and constant throughout the entire respiratory cycle. This results in a constant flow pattern and equal cycles of inhalation and exhalation. Steadiness is very important as interruptions of flow, such as jerkiness and pauses, directly affect autonomic balance. A related technique is 2:1 breathing, in which the exhalation is twice as long as the inhalation. If exhalation is twice as long as inhalation, the parasympathetic system is subtly but directly stimulated more than the sympathetic. This results in a slight dominance of parasympathetic tone, and thus a state of relaxation.

One of the most important breathing exercises in yoga is alternate nostril breathing, or channel purification. This exercise expands a person's conscious control over respiratory motion and increases vital capacity. It is a simple, straightforward exercise that leads directly to balanced autonomic tone. Vital capacity is also increased by the practice of a variety of "bellows" exercises. These are forceful exhalations and/or inhalations designed to cleanse the lungs and increase lung resiliency.

The most subtle practice is breath awareness. This involves focusing the attention on the base of the bridge of the nostrils and simply attending to the "feeling" and the quality of the breath. This is distinctly a perceptual practice, that leads to increased awareness of internal mental events. This intensive perceptual practice gradually leads to the conscious awareness and control of the subtle patterns of energy. This control is the goal of the practice of pranayama.

The relationship between the body, breath, and mind illustrates the comprehensive view of yoga science. While Western science and medicine constantly refer to the mind/body relationship, they do not explain the mechanism for interaction in this relationship. This is particularly true of current theories of stress. Even those theories that are psychological in nature, such as the psychophysiologic and psychoanalytic, fail to fully explain the mechanism for interaction in the relationship between mind and body. In yoga science, however, this relationship is explained by the sheath of energy that intervenes between the physical and mental sheaths. Energy is recognized as the link between mind and body, and breath is the major vehicle for this energy. In yoga science, there is a detailed analysis of energy structures and patterns. In fact, the science of pranayama is considered to be a vast and distinct body of knowledge.[34]

Although the breath and the energy sheath are major factors in understanding stress, or autonomic imbalance, it is the central nervous system that provides the primary control for autonomic functioning. In the next section, we will explore the role of the manomaya kosha, or mental sheath, in the comprehensive framework of human dysfunction, or stress, that is found in yoga science.

The Central Nervous System

The definition of stress as autonomic imbalance, while logically consistent and very powerful, also implies that this physiological manifestation of imbalance is the end result of more subtle events. Our definition of stress is not a final answer, but rather a starting place from which to explore inwardly toward the more central and more subtle determining events. Thus, our definition follows the introspective, empirical method of yoga science, moving from the gross to the more subtle.

The work done by Western scientists in exploring physiological processes is both sophisticated and extensive, but limited. The problem lies not in the factual knowledge, but rather in the relational organization of that knowledge, and in the mechanistic anad reductionistic blindness to underlying causal realities. In this section we will seek to gain a further understanding of the definition of stress as autonomic imbalance. Within the physical sheath, the principal regulatory system is the nervous system. The peripheral autonomic system is influenced indirectly by the other peripheral system, the sensory-motor system, and directly regulated by the central nervous system. Beginning with the peripheral system, it is well-known that there is a close relationship between motor activity and sympathetic arousal. What generally goes unnoticed is the impact of sensory-motor activation on autonomic functioning. Constant motor activity and sensory input have a strong impact on sympathetic tone.

For example, the constant level of noise and the hectic pace of life in New York City leads to a chronic imbalance. People don't even realize they are tired until they leave the constant stimulation. To understand this influence, we must go to the higher-order regulatory system, the central nervous system, and in particular the Reticular Activating System (RAS) located in the brain stem. The RAS is thought to regulate "the overall degree of central nervous system activity, including control of wakefulness and sleep, and control of at least part of our ability to direct attention toward specific areas of our conscious mind."[35]

The RAS is stimulated by sensory activation. In fact, almost any type of sensory signal can activate the RAS, and this activation is referred to as the "arousal reaction."

The most important or powerful activation occurs from the sensory signals of pain and movement. There is also activation of the RAS from cerebral activity. There are an exceedingly large number of nerve fibers that pass from the motor regions of the cerebral cortex to the RAS. Consequently, we find that motor activity, in particular, is associated with wakefulness. It is important to understand, however, that intense activity of any other part of the cerebrum can also activate the RAS and, consequently, cause a high level of wakefulness or alertness.

Stimulation of the RAS increases autonomic activity throughout the body. There is an increase in sympathetic activity that causes the release of epinephrine. This, in turn, has a reciprocal effect on the brain stem, further enhancing its activity and increasing wakefulness. Thus, increases in the intensity and frequency of the action of the sensory systems, as well as increased motor activity through activated regions of the cerebral cortex, all lead to increased RAS activity. This in turn leads to increased sympathetic tone and degrees of wakefulness. Thus, incoming sensory input and motor activity play a significant role in autonomic arousal.

High levels of sensory input, and/or constant motor activity, can lead to autonomic imbalance. It is particularly important to recognize that adaptation to high levels of sensory input does not necessarily mean there is no imbalance of the autonomic system. In fact, all evidence points to continuous imbalance, and consequently, stress.

As we can see, regulation of the peripheral sensory-motor system can influence RAS activity, and influence autonomic balance. If the sensory-motor system is not regulated, then the input through the RAS to the autonomic system is also unregulated, resulting in autonomic imbalance, or stress. In yoga science, there are specific practices to regulate sensory activity, called *pratyahara,* or sensory regulation, as well as specific methods for regulating postural and motor responses, such as hatha yoga and, in particular, the corpse posture. Some of these practices will be discussed in other chapters of this anthology.

Autonomic functioning, although stimulated by the RAS, is under the direct control of another substructure of the central nervous system called the limbic system. The limbic system is a grouping of brain structures directly above the brain stem. It consists "of sub-cortical structures, such as the hypothalamus and adjacent areas . . . older portions of the cerebral cortex that are located on the medial and ventral portions of the cerebral hemispheres. . . ."[36] The limbic system directly regulates autonomic functioning, and is responsible for the so-called vegetative functions, such as regulation of arterial pressure, body fluid balance, electrolyte content of body fluids, gastrointestinal activity, and many internal secretions of the endocrine glands.

The various neural structures and glands that comprise the limbic system are also responsible for much of the emotional response in man—so much so that the limbic system is often referred to as the "seat of emotions" in humans. Through direct control of the autonomic endocrine systems, the limbic system is the major regulatory agency for the psychosomatic effects in the body. Its major structure is the hypothalamus, which not only regulates both sympathetic and parasympathetic functioning, but also provides excitation to the Reticular Activating System.

The "highest" brain center is the cerebral cortex, which is responsible for the intellectual functions of the brain. It is here that thoughts, images, memory, and perceptual organization and interpretation primarily take place, along with the related motor responses. While the connections are complex and not completely understood, it is increasingly clear that cortical activities are the primary determinants of both limbic activity and RAS functioning.

Whether or not an alarm response is activated is determined primarily by events in the cerebral cortex that are related to our perceptual and thinking process:

"If the external stimulus is brief and if we do not extend activation in the cortex by ruminating on the threatening event, the associated autonomic response mediated in the hypothalamus will be brief. This might involve a mild increase in sympathetic discharge (with perhaps some increased adrenal hormone release), but without major activation of the emotions or the hormonal systems associated with the pituitary gland. In such a case, overall functioning can return very quickly to a balanced, relaxed state. If the external stimulus is maintained because one cannot resolve a problem (or through persistent worry), then increasing degrees of sympathetic arousal can result which involve and reinforce greater degrees of emotional intensity. Then the pituitary, thyroid, and adrenal cortex responses become involved."[37]

And later on:

"Autonomic functioning is controlled mainly by the events that occur in the cerebral cortex, the part of the brain that organizes perceptual data and provides the context by which we interpret our world. *Thus the primary source of stress is not the external environment: it is the emotional and perceptual factors which form our basic personality.* The greatest source of hypothalamic arousal comes from our own cerebral cortex in response to repetitive thought patterns, constant worries, and apprehensions about unresolved past, present, or future events which are associated with potentially painful or negative consequences in our lives.

Stress, then, is a physiological response to one's mental activities; it is the way we think about a situation that determines whether or not we will generate it."[38]

Thus, we have a hierarchical, interpenetrating system of regulatory control in the physical sheath that begins in the periphery and ascends to a central structure (the brain), which is hierarchically structured. The ultimate potential of control lies in the cerebral cortex, the control room of mental events.

It is within the subtle mental sheath, the manomaya kosha, that the so-called intellectual activities occur that are expressed through cortical activity. In the following section we will continue our development of this framework of stress by exploring a more subtle layer of human functioning—the mental sheath.

Stress and the Mental Sheath

At this, the third level or sheath of human functioning, the focus shifts to the mind and its various functions. Although there are important sources of stress, such as diet and environmental factors (for example, air and noise pollution or weather extremes) that impact the body without the necessity of determinate mental activity, the single most significant source of stress is that resulting from the activation of an alarm response (fight or flight or the possum response). This alarm response is keyed to the perception of a threat. It is irrelevant whether or not the threat actually exists—only that the individual perceives it as existing. The anticipated harm may not even be perceived as a present danger, but may in fact be a memory of a past danger, or even a fantasy of danger. Whether perceived in the usual sense, fantasized, or recalled, the process that leads to physiological activation is a mental one and must be understood within a truly psychological context. Sophisticated analysis of neural activity, such as electroencephalography or biochemical analysis of glandular secretions, while useful in expanding our knowledge of brain functioning, does not give us insight into the significant functional capacity or dynamic interactions of the mind. What is needed is direct perceptual awareness of the mind and its activities. This requires an understanding of the subtleties of the mind and its interaction with the brain/body complex.

This direct perceptual knowledge requires a sophisticated and effective system of introspection. For example, one of the greatest sources of stress is the constant stream of thoughts, images, and sensations that the famous psychologist, William James, called the "stream of consciousness." We often glorify this inner chatter by calling it "thinking," but often there is very little "thought" behind it at all. It is this inner chatter, both conscious and unconscious, that is the source of a great deal of our stress.

When we examine this inner dialogue, we find that the mind has the capacity to live in the future, to focus on the present, or to relive the past. We can remember what we did last week, anticipate what will happen tomorrow, or focus on what is occurring now. The mind moves with ease through time, since time, at least as we experience it, is created by the mind in order to analyze sensory data.

The brain, however, being a physical object, is far more limited. It operates only in what we may call "real time," or the present. The brain is not the mind, but rather the control mechanism through which the mind operates on this level of being. The brain is best understood as a sophisticated biocomputer that is an enormous transducer, translating the subtle energy of the mind into the biochemical/bioelectrical energy of the body.

When there is a thought or image in the mind, the brain is already busy translating that thought or image into physical energy. It prepares the body to perform the actions inherent in that thought or image. For example, if I am thinking of having a conflict with someone, my body is *now* being prepared to take the necessary action even though the conflict is purely in my mind, and at this point, purely imaginary. The greater my emotional involvement, the greater the changes in my body. Or I can remember a terrible thing that happened last week (or last year, or even years ago) and create a great deal of change in my body.

This imbalance between the past-and-future thinking mind and the present-oriented brain leads directly to autonomic imbalance, and thus generates a state of stress. When mind and body (brain) are coordinated, imbalance does not occur. This often happens when we become absorbed in a task we are doing. Our experience is then fulfilling even though we may work very hard. This experience can be contrasted with a circumstance in which we didn't have much to do, but we sat and worried about what might happen. When our mind is scattered with worries, regrets, and other disturbances, we find our bodies disturbed; we are tense and worn-out, and feel very dissatisfied.

One immediate tool for focusing and clearing the mind of this inner chatter is breath awareness. Breath awareness is becoming aware of the feeling of coolness of the inhalation and the slight touch of warmth of the exhalation at the opening of the nostrils. The focus is on feeling the breath, a perceptual act, rather than thinking about the breath. This peceptual awareness immediately establishes a calmness in the mind; the inner chatter is quieted, the breath naturally slows and becomes more even (and in turn brings balance to the autonomic nervous system) and the body relaxes. Since there are no more "instructions" coming from the mind/brain, the poor body can relax. The body's natural state is one of relaxation. It becomes agitated because the mind becomes agitated. The deeper the calm of the mind, the more profound is the state of rest for the body.

This is why the practice of meditation, which is deep inner concentration, brings about so many profound and positive changes to the body. Although still in its infancy, western research on states of inner concentration (often mistakenly referred to as meditation) suggest that meditation leads to a more balanced, stable, and relaxed physiology, as well as a less anxious, more fulfilled mental state.

There are many such subtleties to the mind/body (brain) interaction that have direct impact on whether or not we are under stress. One significant factor is concentration. Concentration is not a one dimensional act, but rather consists of a blend of varying dimensions that determine not only the form and quality of the concentrative state, but also the consequences. For example, one important dimension of concentration is the underlying motivation dimension of positive interest (e.g., curiosity) or negative interest (e.g., fear).

When the mind perceives a threat and activates an alarm response, the mind becomes concentrated (or preoccupied) with the threat. The greater the threat, the more intense the concentration. However, this form of concentration is all too often a disaster. It involves increasing states of physiological readiness, an increasing restriction of one's awareness to the "problem" (threat). That is itself a "closing down" of the mind called "tunnel vision," which excludes more and better possibilities of actions and solutions. The consequences of this state of concentration are increased imbalance and stress, increasingly rigid and inappropriate behaviors, and loss of personal effectiveness.

On the other hand, a different quality and form of concentration occurs in the absence of threat and is the result of one's positive interest. This concentration is characterized by a calm, focused mind. During this state of concentration, awareness is actually expanded, more perceptual knowledge is available for conscious and even unconscious use, and creativity is stimulated. It is characterized by and facilitates a state of inner balance and leads to a profound relaxation in the body. Stress is physiologically incompatible with this state of being.

Other dimensions are equally important in the quality and form of concentration. Briefly, these are the level of energy (high or low, increasing or decreasing), the direction or orientation (internal or external), the quality of focus (one-pointed or dissipated), and the time orientation. Another major factor is one's conscious skill at regulating these dimensions and the concentrative states. All of these interact to determine the duality and form of concentration, and as a consequence, play a direct role in whether or not one suffers from stress.

There are many other aspects of the mind and the mind/brain interaction that affect our capacity to regulate ourselves and be free of stress. Our positive and negative emotions, attitudes, and beliefs, the various levels of mind, and much more are all involved. The key to their understanding, regulation, and use is direct experiential knowledge. The failure of Western psychology and medicine to provide a scientific and practical basis for successful self-regulation and self-transformation is that they lack a sophisticated system of introspection that can be used to gain the direct, experiential knowledge and the consequent holistic understanding of human functioning that is based on that direct experience.

The direct, systematic, experiential base of yoga science has led to the formulation of a psychology that is radically different in major aspects from the materialistic and reductionistic systems of Western science and in particular, Western psychology. Two primary and significant differences are the recognition in yoga psychology of the primacy and irreducibility of non-material realities and the material reality of mind as separate from and superior to the body (brain).

In the reductionistic systems of psychology (and science), consciousness is "nothing but" a reactivity of the physical structure called the brain and is thus directly dependent upon neurological structure and function. Obviously, from a materialistic viewpoint, if there is no brain there is no consciousness. The term "mind," long in disfavor in "knowledgeable scientific circles," is an ambiguous term roughly representing the organizational capacity and function of the brain and related neurological structures (fig. 5). Often the terms "consciousness" and "mind" are used as equivalent concepts, with little or no discrimination between them.

Figure 5

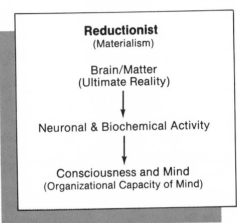

Reductionist
(Materialism)

Brain/Matter
(Ultimate Reality)

↓

Neuronal & Biochemical Activity

↓

Consciousness and Mind
(Organizational Capacity of Mind)

Probably the clearest statement of strict reductionistic belief is given by astronomer Carl Sagan in *The Dragons of Eden*, in which he states: "My fundamental premise about the brain is that its workings—what we sometimes call mind—are a consequence of its anatomy and physiology, and nothing more."[39] It is interesting to note that Sagan, after examining the "clear trend in the recent history of biology and because there is not a shred of evidence to support it," will not even entertain any hypothesis concerning something "inhabiting the matter of the body made of quite different stuff called mind" (note the dependency on material matter—i.e., "stuff").[40] In short, we have a modern phraseology for the old materialist saw concerning the surgeon cutting up the body and not finding the soul.

An alternative Western view is found in the recent work of such eminent brain researchers as Wilder Penfield,[41] Sir John Eccles,[42] Karl Pribram,[43] and particularly Roger Sperry.[44] Sperry states explicitly that mental events control physical events, and that consciousness is an emergent property of the brain, with capacities that are greater than the sum of the capacities of the parts (the brain) involved. Barbara Brown in *Supermind*[45] points out (in direct contradiction to Sagan) that "the research data of the sciences themselves point much more strongly toward the existence of a mind-more-than-brain than they do toward mere mechanical brain action." Mind is seen here as an emergent property, with status not only independent of, but even superior to the brain, or matter (see fig. 6). Consciousness, however, is still a quality of the mind-brain interaction.

We must also assume (although it has not been directly discussed) that even those who support this apparent Cartesian dualism of mind-matter (brain) do not intend that either mind or consciousness continues on once its matter base (the brain and biological energy) is extinguished. Consequently, in Western systems, even in those which now distinguish mind from brain, consciousness is relegated to the position of being the expression and reactivity

Figure 6

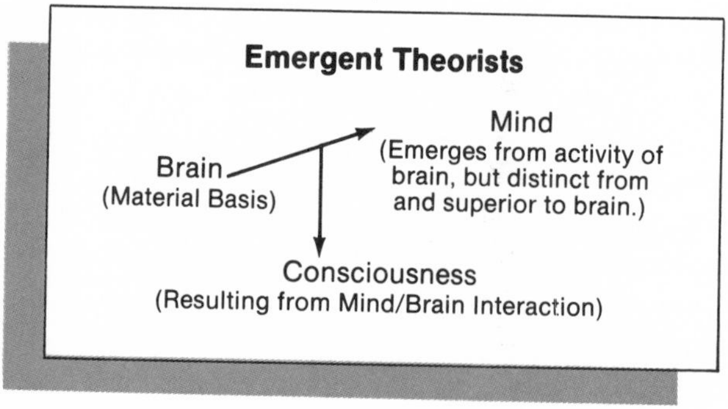

Emergent Theorists

Brain (Material Basis) → Mind (Emerges from activity of brain, but distinct from and superior to brain.)

Consciousness (Resulting from Mind/Brain Interaction)

of biological energy in the physical structure. Consciousness is born with the body and dies with the body.

In yoga psychology, however, consciousness (cit) is the fundamental reality underlying being and/or identity and the material world. This pure consciousness is dissociated from mind and matter, and is what Merrell-Wolff refers to as *Consciousness without an Object*.[46] It is a non-material reality that is not subject to time and space and thus to cause/effect relationships. Being non-material, it is also non-logical and cannot be proven or deduced through logical methods, as for instance, research methods designed to investigate material realities, or the surgeon's knife. However, its validity and reality can be ultimately established through direct experience. The experience of pure consciousness without an object is, in fact, considered to be the ultimate, or perfect (i.e., unlimited) experience. According to the yoga science, consciousness is the source of all manifestation. This one unchanging reality, when regarded as the unchanging principle of consciousness in its formless, unlimited essence is called Shiva. This is the universal consciousness without an object. The power of consciousness to limit itself and thus manifest form, to create and project the universe from out of itself, is called Shakti. Pure consciousness does not exist without this power: this power cannot potentiate out of non-consciousness. Consciousness and the consciousness-power are one and the same.

All energy, called prana, is the expression of the power of consciousness and will take one of two forms: energy appearing as an agent is called *cit-shakti*, energy appearing as a material or instrument is called *maya-shakti*. Energy itself is not consciousness, nor is it Shakti. It is, rather, the signature of consciousness and is manifest through the inherent power (Shakti) of consciousness.

There are three interactive tendencies inherent in the operation of Shakti that determine the outcome of the operation, depending on which tendency is dominant. These three tendencies are referred to as the *gunas,* and are named *sattva, rajas,* and *tamas.* Sattva (essence) is the revealing tendency, the tendency of Shakti to lead back to pure consciousness, or Shiva. Rajas (energy or activity) is the energizing tendency, the tendency of Shakti to activate. Tamas (inertia) is the veiling tendency, the tendency of Shakti to imitation. All three gunas are active at all times, but one will dominate and lead to a particular manifestation.

When consciousness is enveloped or acted upon by its power or Shakti with the revealing tendency, sattva, predominant, that which becomes manifest is mind, or antahkarana, the "inner instrument." When consciousness is acted upon (enveloped) by Shakti with the energizing tendency, rajas, predominant, that which is manifested is the life force. When consciousness is enveloped by Shakti with the veiling tendency, tamas, predominant, that which becomes manifest is matter in the Western sense.

Thus, using this basic relational framework of consciousness, mind, and matter (fig. 7), we can now understand mind to be a limited form of consciousness, an energy field with extension into time and space. As a form of energy, mind is a material reality and not consciousness itself, which pervades the form. Mind is a subtle form of matter (energy) and is referred to as "radiant matter." It is a finite material reality, with various capacities and functions, but dependent upon and subservient to consciousness.

Matter is also a manifestation of the power of consciousness. Although mind is a very subtle energy field, matter is a very gross energy field. Both are material realities, formed from energy. Mind is a limited form of consciousness as a finite subject, while matter is a limited form of consciousness as the finite object. Both mind and matter result from the power of limitation of consciousness. Whatever appears as a limitation of consciousness

Figure 7

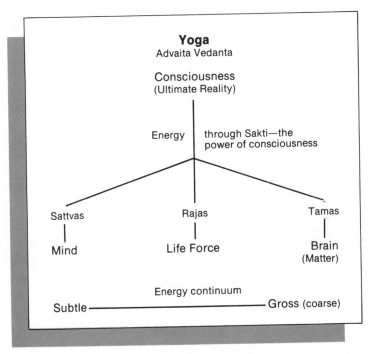

can only be temporal, since only consciousness itself is universal and unlimited. Any limitation of consciousness, being only temporal, is thus considered to be not consciousness, or rather, unconscious, though universal consciousness is still the underlying source. Thus, both mind and matter (brain) are objects of consciousness. As we shall see later, this is a factor that has considerable importance in gaining accurate, objective, and direct knowledge of mental events. This power of consciousness to limit itself is often called maya-shakti.

Mind and matter originate from the same universal reality and by the same power, Shakti. Between mind and matter, then, there is no essential or qualitative difference, only one of degree, and both are subject to time, space, and causality. Mind, as the more subtle energy, pervades the body and is the more potent force. In yoga psychology, the more subtle the energy form, the greater the potency of the energy form. The body is a greater limitation, a more bound form of energy, and thus not as pervasive or as powerful as the less bound, less limited form called mind. The mind may exist without the body, the body is dependent upon the mind for its support. This relationship is reflected in the yogic statement, "all of the body is in the mind, but not all of the mind is in the body." Obviously, the material base proposed by the reductionistic systems of Western psychology is directly denied in yoga psychology. The causal sequence in yoga psychology begins with consciousness, proceeds through the mind, and then there is the body. The physical structure is the least powerful and the least significant.

This leads to a further significant distinction between reductionistic systems and yoga psychology. In reductionistic systems, there is an absolute separation between "subjective" phenomena (internal mental events) and "objective" phenomena (external events). In other words, the universe of thought and the universe of objects—the "see-touch" world—are qualitatively two separate universes. At best, these two worlds exist in some sort of parallelism, and they interface and interact with each other but remain distinct and separate.

Furthermore, the subjective universe is not considered to have a substantial enough reality to directly quantify, measure, or explore in a "scientific" or objective way. The materialistic bias of Western psychology has led to a denial of the possibility of scientifically studying "subjective" phenomena directly. Since one cannot "objectively" measure, record, systematize, or observe a mental event, then obviously one cannot scientifically study subjective phenomena. Obviously, one cannot have as an object of observation the very internal process that one is using to observe. In plain language, according to Western psychology, direct knowledge of one's own thought processes is not scientifically valid because we are subject to tremendous distortion when we observe ourselves. The mind cannot objectively study itself.

Consequently, heroic efforts have been made in Western psychology to study subjective phenomena indirectly by "objectifying" subjective data. Efforts such as projective tests, scaling methodologies, personality inventories, diagnostic interviews, process analysis, imagery and symbolism analysis, dream analysis, and behavior analysis are just a few of the main strategies developed to indirectly measure and thus come to understand the inner reality. In fact, entire systems of psychology have been developed in order to bypass the "black box" and its seemingly ephemeral contents.

The consequences of the strong materialistic, Newtonian bias in Western science and psychology has been to deny the possibility of directly studying internal mental processes. Obviously, the mind, if it really did exist, could only be known indirectly or by studying one's behavior, whether it was test behavior, dream behavior, or global personality behaviors and traits.

Thus, if you really wanted to know yourself, you had to enlist the aid of someone who could help you interpret these behaviors, or perhaps give you psychological tests. Direct knowledge was, and is, considered to be extremely suspect, subject to considerable distortion. In other words, if you wanted to know the inner realities of yourself, you had to pay attention to the external symptoms and behaviors. It is as if by looking outward, you will somehow see inward. With this sort of reasoning, it's not at all surprising that there is so much confusion in our Western psychological systems.

This is a very real problem in Western psychology. Direct, experiential knowledge free from perceptual distortion is generally not available in Western reductionist systems. Western psychology has never developed a scientific, systematic system of introspection, nor has it developed any systematic study of mind or consciousness. In fact, it has precluded the validity of such a system of knowledge largely because of unexamined materialist assumptions concerning the nature of consciousness and mind.

Conversely, yoga psychology has developed a systematic, verifiable, and empirical science of introspection. It is not the introspection used in the early days of psychophysics, nor the subjective reporting being utilized today. Rather, it is the systematic expansion of conscious awareness that has its basis in the direct, conscious experience of non-material consciousness. In this state of expanded awareness, objective knowledge about the mind, its contents, and functioning, is available to the individual. This direct experiential knowledge leads to the conscious control over the mind and matter. The more one is able to "step outside the mind" and establish one's identity or sense-of-I-ness within pure consciousness, the more one can understand clearly and control the mind.

This control and understanding gives us a whole new perspective on managing stress. First of all, we are able to understand the mental patterns that shape our perceptions and ignite our habitual emotional reactions, thereby maintaining the inner habits by which we create stress for ourselves. Secondly, we have control in terms of choosing to change these mental causes of stress. A correct understanding of the nature of mind and the direct experience of witnessing one's own mental flow are, of course, prerequisites for managing stress at this most essential level. Any program of stress management that is not based on such an understanding and experience is superficial. Such a program is simply not getting at the root causes of stress.

When one does begin to work at this essential mental level, however, it is possible to develop a more consistent balance, an enduring harmony, and an ultimate freedom from stress.

CHAPTER 10
Perception and Stress

John R. Harvey, Ph.D.

The occurrence, intensity, and duration of the stress response are determined by our perception of events. When we consider this fact we often attempt to reduce stress by modifying our perceptions. Typically this is done by changing the thought patterns, that is, the cognitive-evaluative portion of perception. Our underlying assumption is usually that the perceptual process, the activity of the senses, is generally an autonomous and objective mechanism. Yet with careful analysis we can see that the process of perception is dynamic, creative, and subjective. By understanding the perceptual process and learning to regulate and transform it we have another access route to managing the stress response. Let us begin to develop this path of stress reduction by reviewing some basic considerations about the nature of perception.

We continually make contact with the world around us through our sense organs. An ever-shifting pattern of images, sounds, smells, tastes, and tactile sensations comes into our mind to shape our ongoing experience of life. To some degree we even organize our life around perceptual experiences, seeking out what is pleasant and avoiding what is repugnant. Loud, shrill noises, grotesque sights, and unpleasant smells have an immediate effect on our emotional state, producing fear, anxiety, disgust, or sadness. We consciously and unconsciously avoid these stimuli. On the other hand, we may devote considerable time, effort, and money to procuring tasty food, rich fragrances, and pleasing sights, which at least initially create more positive emotional states. We live in a world of sensory experience; our emotions, our decisions, and our thoughts all occur in response to our perceptions.

Considering the tremendous impact of sensory experience in our life, it is not surprising that many of the ancient systems of psychology examined this topic very thoroughly. These ancient systems that were concerned with self-development and self-realization, such as yoga psychology, noted that understanding and mastery of the senses were vital topics. The role of perception in emotional health and mental well-being was carefully scrutinized in the yogic tradition.

In this chapter we will examine the concept of perception in yoga psychology and look at the practical guidelines this science set forth to achieve mastery of perception. However, before we journey further into the territory of yoga psychology, let us examine what is already widely known about perception.

Because we live in a technological world of machines it is easy for us to make mechanistic assumptions regarding our sense organs. We view them as little machines, objective and mechanical in their function, capable of occasional glitches and subject to wear and tear and breakdown. We assume that we are equipped with a video recorder, a tape deck, a fragrance meter, touch receptors, and an array of high-fidelity taste receptors. These little sense machines collect data and allow us to piece together a relatively accurate picture of the world around us. We believe that the information brought in is entirely a function of what is "out there." If we change the objective surroundings, we change our sensory input. All these assumptions lead us to a highly objective model of perception, in which we believe the external objects determine what is perceived.

When we reflect on our own experience, however, we find many challenges to this objective model. We all know what it means to look but not really see, to hear but not really listen. It is as if the objects are out there but we don't register or notice their presence. Stop reading for a minute and look carefully around the room. If you look around the room in a fresh manner, you may be surprised at how much you hadn't noticed. Or close your eyes and just listen to all the sounds. Once again, you may be surprised at the wealth of new sounds you become aware of—that is to say, sounds that are new to you because you are now directing your attention to them. Thus, attention influences what we perceive and to some degree how it affects us.

Another important point is the effect of mood on our perceptions. When we feel depressed or agitated, we often find that nothing looks good. Everything around us may seem grey, ugly, and in a state of decay. We may have little taste for food, and all smells may seem unpleasant. Every little sound may grate on our nerves. This contrasts sharply with how everything appears to us when we feel good: then the world and everything in it looks, smells, and feels wonderful; even the rumble of trucks and cars has a special music to it. So it seems that a second internal factor, our emotional state, also affects our perceptions.

Our culture and environment also play a role in shaping our perceptual experience. We come to share perceptions with our social group. These perceptions fit our environment. A dramatic illustration is given by Philip Zimbardo and Floyd Ruch in their book *Psychology and Life.*[1] They describe an experience of the anthropologist Colin Turnbull, who studied the African Pygmies. The Pygmies inhabit a thick tropical forest where vision is limited and the natives rely extensively on auditory cues. Turnbull relates the following anecdote about his taking a hunter, Kenge, out to the open plain:

> Kenge looked over the plains and down to where a herd of about a hundred buffalo were grazing some miles away. He asked me what kind of insects they were, and I told him they were buffalo, twice as big as the forest buffalo known to him. He laughed loudly and told me not to tell such stupid stories, and asked me again what kind of insects they were. He then talked to himself, for want of more intelligent company, and tried to liken the buffalo to the various beetles and ants with which he was familiar.
>
> He was still doing this when we got into the car and drove down to where the animals were grazing. He watched them getting larger and larger, and though he was as courageous as any Pygmy, he moved over and sat close to me and muttered that it was witchcraft.
>
> Finally, when he realized that they were real buffalo he was no longer afraid, but what puzzled him still was why they had been so small, and whether they really had been small and had so suddenly grown larger, or whether it had been some kind of trickery.

Kenge apparently had acquired an internal scheme of how things should be according to his cultural and physical environment. He tried to make the new data fit his learned perceptual rules. Many of us may have experienced similar perceptual frustration in a strange or new environment.

Reviewing these points of common experience, we come to the inescapable conclusion that a great many factors influence our internal state and affect our perception: perceptual habits inculcated by our culture and environment can determine how we interpret sensory data; suggestion and social influence can radically affect our perceptions; our mood seems to affect the quality of our perceptions; and we note in everyday experience that attention is a prerequisite for accurately perceiving what's around us.

These factors lead us to the conclusion that perception is not merely determined by the object "out there" but is instead highly influenced by factors within the person perceiving. Thus, it appears that perception is often more subjective than objective. In other words, it is more a function of the person perceiving than of the object perceived. In yoga science, perception is seen as highly subjective, and considerable emphasis is devoted to understanding those internal mechanisms influencing perception. However, before we consider the perspective of yoga science, let us further examine what Western science has discovered regarding perception.

First of all, some issues of terminology must be considered. Western science differentiates between sensation and perception. Sensation deals with the collection of sensory impressions, and tends to emphasize the anatomical structure of the sense organ and the neural pathways. Perception, on the other hand, deals with the subjective experience. Past learning can shape and influence raw sensory data and turn it into a perceptual experience rich in conceptual thinking.

Western scientists are clearly acquainted with the subjective implications of perception and the ultimate difficulty in studying this process. As noted by Peter Milner, "The study of sensory mechanisms involves us in some very difficult problems, verging on the metaphysical."[2] Since Western science feels uncomfortable with the metaphysical, its focus has been more on the sensory processes, neural pathways, and cortical mechanisms involved in sensate functioning.

Research in this area has resulted in fascinating findings regarding the anatomy and capabilities of the senses. For example, the average human has approximately ten thousand taste buds (children have more), while chickens have only twenty-four. A given receptor cell within a taste bud may be active only for a few days before it degenerates and its place is taken by another receptor cell. As another example, the sense of smell is thought to be one of the keenest senses in a human: there are approximately thirty million receptors per nostril. Sniffing radically increases the flow of air over the receptor cells, thereby increasing the olfactory sensitivity.

Sight is probably the most studied of the senses. The structure of the eye resembles a camera, with a lens that focuses and a retina that catches the images. The eye has been found to have amazing capacities and can differentiate between seven million different shades of color. The sense of touch is similarly complex, and includes not only the skin senses of touch, pressure, pain, temperature, itch, and vibration, but also the internal body senses of joint position, muscle tension, and visceral state.

When one considers these various sensations and the stupendous number of sense receptors throughout the body, the wealth of information that is potentially available is amazing. Our sense of hearing depends on the smallest bones in the body, which together with an intricate fluid system capture an astounding range of vibrations. The ear of the average young person is sensitive to frequencies in the range of from twenty hertz to twenty thousand hertz.

Because all of these sensory systems are so complex, each is a field of study in itself. In a reductionist/materialistic view of existence, such as is predominant in the modern world, a sensory system is a more "real" and therefore less troublesome area of study than the subjective aspects of perception. An exclusive study of the sensory mechanisms lends itself to a highly objective model of perception and has probably contributed to our popular conception of the senses as little recording machines conveniently placed throughout the body.

In studying the more subjective aspects of perception, Western researchers have long been fascinated with illusions.

These represent ways in which our senses are tricked. Thus, illusions seem to have the promise of giving us insights into the rules that govern perception. Some well-known illusions may be seen in figures 1 and 2. Figure 1 deals with figure and ground, which in this case are reversible. When we see the white area as the figure of a cup it takes on definition and appears nearer and more vivid than it does when we view it as the ground for the two profiles. The tendency to select a salient characteristic or figure reflects a perceptual rule to establish unity and wholeness in our perceptions.

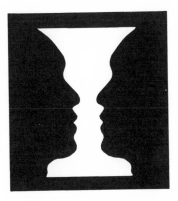

Figure 1

The illusion represented in figure 2 demonstrates the tendency to evaluate things visually based on nearby cues. In this case the angled lines change our sense of distance: segment *a* is actually shorter than segment *b*. Thus, illusions are fascinating, and by apparently bending our perceptual rules they help us to discover these rules.

Western scientists have also studied the more phenomenological aspects of perception. Researchers have attempted to systematically identify the psychological or internal factors that influence our perceptual experience. Foremost among these factors is learning. Perception appears to develop as

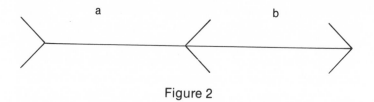

Figure 2

the infant matures. The specific experiences provided by a culture determine the type of perceptual habits that develop in its members.

For example, it has been verified that individuals raised in a culture where reading goes from left to right tend to employ left to right scanning in most situations. However, the opposite is true for individuals trained to read right to left. Another example is the musical scale. Westerners who are trained to hear music built on a scale of half and whole tones tend to think, hear, feel, and hum to themselves utilizing these types of tones. A quite different musical ear and humming pattern is developed in cultures where quarter tones and even micro tones are part of the musical scale.

Other variables affecting perception include values, expectancies, motives, needs, and emotional states. A classic experiment demonstrating the effect of these variables was conducted by hypnotizing subjects, suggesting to them either a financially rich history or a poor history, and then having the subjects adjust a spot of light to match the size of either a nickel, dime, or quarter.[3] Those subjects hypnotized as "poor" made the coin sizes larger than normal, while the "rich" subjects made them smaller. The experimenters concluded that the values and needs established in subjects via hypnotic suggestions affected the size estimates they made.

From a more clinical perspective, projective personality tests such as the Rorschach inkblots have shown that individuals who share emotional states such as depression tend to have similar perceptions in terms of form, color, and movement. Depression, an internal state, influences the way we perceive the world. Depressed individuals, when asked to draw a person, often omit the hands and feet, which is frequently interpreted as a sign of helplessness. Other emotional states such as anxiety, paranoia, and mania also have a strong selective and creative influence on our perception.

These clinical considerations underscore what might be called the "vicious cycle" aspect of stress. For example, if people are confronted with a number of significant personal losses, they may become depressed. The state of depression may then influence their perception so that they are more sensitive to other negative events in their life. Dwelling on these events can easily deepen the depression and make them even more sensitive and more selectively focused on events related to their helpless, frustrated state. Thus, unless we have a method of interrupting this type of vicious cycle, most strong, negative, emotional states associated with stress will tend to influence perception in a manner that actually perpetuates excessive stress responding and makes us more vulnerable to other stressors.

Let us organize our review of perception by considering three models of the perceptual process. The first is predominantly objective and is related to psychophysics. The emphasis here is on the physical stimulus and the accompanying receptor and neural pathway functioning. Misperceptions are seen as quirks and errors in which the senses misread the objective data. This view is essentially materialistic and implies that reality is "out there" in the material world.

A second model might be labeled as "objective, with subjective shadings." This model accepts the findings of psychophysics in terms of the mechanics of the senses. However, it takes a different approach to errors or illusions, which are seen as indicating that there are a number of factors that lawfully influence the psychological or internal aspects of perception. In this model there are certain lawful relationships governing the object, the senses, and the internal processing.

A third model is somewhat more subjective and less objective. Here, it is assumed that perception is an experience. Given this starting point, one tries to make some sense of the various objective and subjective factors. This third model is somewhat less rigorously scientific and more purely psychological. Adherents of this model seek simultaneously to utilize the hard facts about sensory mechanics and to pay credence to the vast world of subjectivity. The great difficulty here is that there are no parameters to define internal experience.

Yogic Theory of Perception

Yoga psychology presents us with a fourth perspective on perception. This one is radically subjective. It is so different from other modern approaches that upon initial exposure it may be hard to accept. Yet this yogic viewpoint carries with it a number of potent implications for therapy, self-development, mental harmony, and for managing stress. The key concept in yoga is the activity of the mind. Perception occurs when mind reaches out to the world of objects through the sense organs, gathers impressions, and creates experience. Accordingly, it is our state of mind that determines our perceptions. The sense organs are the apertures through which the mind flows out. The type of sense organ determines the manner in which the mind moves out, in the same manner that different shapes cut in a cloth allow different patterns of light to shine through.

According to yoga science there are actually fourteen sense organs. These consist of five senses of knowledge, five senses of action, and four internal senses, or aspects of the mind. The five knowledge, or cognitive senses are the ones we are familiar with: sight, touch, smell, taste, and hearing. They are called "knowledge" senses because they define the manner in which we know about the world around us. The action senses concern the manner in which we act upon the world and function physically. These five are speech, grasp, locomotion, evacuation, and generation.

The most important senses are those making up the "inner instrument," or mind. Mind is the dynamic force in perceptual experience. As Swami Akhilananda notes, "According to Indian psychologists it is the mind that reaches out to the objective world through the sense organs and nervous system, drawing the sensations and impressions through them and unifying the experiences gathered into coherent information or knowledge."[4]

The internal organ, mind, is thought to have four distinct functions: *manas,* the sensory-motor mind; *chitta,* the memory bank; *ahamkara,* the ego-sense; and *buddhi,* the decisive intellect. Each perception we have is influenced by each of these components of mind. Perception occurs when the mind travels or moves out in the form of a thought wave, or *vritti.* The thought wave then grasps the object in its wholeness. The object is apprehended in its totality by the thought waves from the mind: the thought waves travel out, envelop the object, and assume its shape. Thus, consciousness, as reflected in the mind, has traveled out and illuminated the object.

A careful sequential analysis of perception allows us to say that the first step involves the mind moving out to apprehend the object. Then manas, the sensory-motor component of the mind, inquires as to whether it is an object or not: if so, which one, and so on. Manas engages in a kind of automatic cataloging activity. Ahamkara, the I-sense, checks to see if the cataloged percept fits with the assumed sense of self. If not, modification of the percept may take place. Simultaneously chitta, the memory bank, associates the perception with previous experiences, thereby stimulating an automatic emotion or motor response. The perceptual experience is now fully formed.

Depending on the level of awareness, a response to the perception may be initiated. With less awareness, the response will be regulated by manas with input from the I-sense and from the memory bank. Thus, the response will be largely conditioned by and consistent with one's assumed sense of self and past conditioning. With more awareness, the data is presented to buddhi, the decisive and more luminous component of mind. Here a decision employing both rational power and creative intuition is made and a response initiated. When this occurs, both the decision and the response are likely to break the stress cycle. A decision facilitated by buddhi is likely to be based on inner awareness and a more objective, unattached view of events.

The more that buddhi is involved in perception, the more spontaneous and insightful the perception is. Our level of awareness influences what and how we perceive. With limited awareness, we perceive in an automatic and stereotyped manner and our responses are automatic. This is the experience of seeing without truly seeing and hearing without really hearing. Real seeing and hearing occur when the discriminative function of mind is engaged; then we see patterns within patterns and hear sounds within sounds. The light of consciousness is reflected in all that we perceive.

Our level of consciousness profoundly influences what we see, feel, hear, taste, and touch. Normally it is the nature of mind to constantly move out into the sensory world. We seek experiences of pleasure again and again. In an effort to avoid discomfort we also scan the environment for sources of pain. Our pleasure-pain attachments dictate how we look at the world.

Our attachments are a function of who we assume we are. Pain and pleasure are largely relative and unique to our self-organization. If we are highly competitive, then we constantly look and listen for evidence of our achievement;

if we are paranoid, we look for enemies; if we are manic, we look for new projects; and if we are spiritually inclined, our mind seeks out manifestations of God's creativity. Thus our inner world, our level of consciousness, selectively creates the world we perceive.

These ideas on the nature of perception stem from a careful study of the mind. The ancient yogis observed the workings of their minds and discovered the roles of the four functions of mind, as well as the roles of awareness and consciousness. They realized that to ultimately regulate perception, one must work internally. In this way the yogis have provided us with a procedure for breaking the stress cycle.

Our experience of life may be transformed by working with our inner instrument, the mind. There are many avenues of intervention. Anything affecting our state of mind will affect our perceptions. Much of what is done in yoga is to decondition or break out of the automatic ways of perceiving. For example, consider what happens when you do a very brief meditation in a familiar environment. Before the meditation you selectively perceive certain aspects of the environment and ignore others. After the meditation the environment may seem different. You may now actually see the pattern on the wallpaper, feel the texture of the furniture, and hear sounds that you hadn't noticed before. You have changed the state of your mind and have thereby changed your perceptions.

In explaining such changes, yoga psychology describes three forces that are known as the *gunas,* or the three aspects of nature, that make up all phenomena. The three are known as *sattva, rajas,* and *tamas.* The sattva guna is the factor of lightness, balance, and harmony. When we meditate, we make our mind more sattvic, and the mental energy is more balanced. Therefore our perceptions are more sattvic. We begin to see more clearly the light, the luminescence, and the essential patterns that unite things and bring them together.

The rajasic mode is one of activity, reaching out, and involvement. When our perception is rajasic, our mind is pulled further and further into the pleasure-pain attachment around us, and we tend to become emotionally involved with events and things. Finally, the tamasic mode is the heavy, depressed, dense, sad, and dark mode. When the mind is in this condition, everything seems to be negative, in disrepair and decay, and to be tinged with grey.

The sattvic mode is characteristic of buddhi, the higher mind. As we create more and more awareness, as we develop more fully our rational and intuitive powers, we begin to reflect the sattvic guna. This influences the way we see and experience the world.

Utilizing the perspective of the gunas, we can consider the effect of certain stimuli on perceptual balance. If we eat stimulating, rajasic food it will make us active, nervous, and distractible. Similarly, if we eat tamasic food—food that is overcooked, old, impure, and heavy—our mind becomes tamasic, heavy, lazy, and inert, and our perception follows suit. On the other hand, when our diet is light, pure, nourishing, and artfully prepared, and when we consume it in an uplifting manner, then we set the stage for an entirely different way of perceiving the world around us. We become sensitive to beauty, truth, and the potential for growth in all things.

The senses are a means to enjoy life. But in yoga this does not mean merely enjoying the material aspects of the world. The yogi uses his senses to perceive the ideal aspects in all things. To the completely trained or enlightened yogi, the phenomenal world is a reflection and affirmation of a higher spiritual reality. The disciplined mind enjoys the image of divine creation. Such a disciplined mind is only possible when one experiences the truth of that ultimate reality that resides within.

Purification of the Senses

In the preceding section we discussed several approaches aimed at maintaining a balanced sensory-mental functioning. We noted some ways in which we can avoid creating imbalance. However, there are further practices in which one works to purify the senses. Here the issue is not just one of health but is instead a question of the more advanced steps required on the path to Self-realization. Under normal conditions the mind is constantly pulled outward toward sensory experiences. Mental energy flows out through the sensory channels and we experience various forms of attachment, aversion, and attraction. We can readily observe and experience the way sensory experience affects us if we take a walk down a busy street in a large city. While walking, we may notice a derelict who is unkempt, dirty, and drunk curled up in a stairway. As we react, the mind is further emotionally involved in that experience. We begin to think, "Oh, that's terrible. How can a person let himself go like that?" Then we may walk a little further and see someone who is dressed very attractively, and we may wish we looked like that, and begin to question our own appearance. Meanwhile a thousand smells and sounds drift through different levels of our awareness, setting off reactions, thoughts, and feelings. This is typical of our everyday experience: the mind is involved in thousands of little dramas. We identify reality as that which occurs outside of us.

This is similar to the functioning of a person caught up in the stress cycle. We develop the habit of letting the senses pour out into the environment and, as a result, our mind and emotions constantly experience ups and downs, pleasures and pain. The negative emotional reactions increase our overall stress levels, and the more we see and hear that upsets us, the more we scan the environment for those sounds and sights that upset us, and thus the momentum of stress grows and feeds upon itself.

The ancient yogis were aware that unregulated sensory functioning leads to increased suffering. Their practical and growth-oriented system of psychology recognized that unless there was regulation of the sensory process it would be exceedingly difficult to attain harmony of mind and body. Control of the senses was consequently seen as a crucial aspect of the process of overcoming suffering and moving toward Self-realization. They called this discipline *pratyahara,* which means "sensory withdrawal." Pratyahara is the fifth of eight steps in the system of self-development known as *raja yoga.*

Of the first four steps, the first two, the *yamas* and *niyamas,* deal with the regulation of social behavior and with guidelines for managing our life. The third step, known as *asana,* deals with postures to make the body comfortable and healthy. The energy of prana, the breath, is channelled in the fourth step, known as *pranayama.* Before we can move to steps six through eight—the internal steps of concentration, meditation, and *samadhi*—we must cover the fifth step, *pratyhara,* or sensory withdrawal. To reach these highest stages we must first learn to regulate the tendency of the mind to flow out, to become identified and attached.

Pratyahara is defined in several sutras in Patanjali's *Yoga Sutras.*[5] The Sutras state that when the senses are no longer pulled towards external objects, they are influenced instead by the essential nature of mind. This withdrawal from external objects leads to control or mastery of the senses. In some of the commentaries on these sutras, the metaphor of a queen bee is used. "Just as bees follow the course of the queen bee and rest when the latter rests, so when the mind stops, the senses also stop their activities."[6] With such mastery we are able to utilize and even enjoy sensory experience, but we avoid creating attachment and suffering.

Control of the senses is a profoundly psychological and spiritual phenomenon. It starts with a conscious decision to direct the mind inward. This decision is based on a philosophical understanding that the world "out there" is one of constant flux and change, an understanding that perceiving consciousness within is a useful goal that allows us to experience an enduring inner peace.

Only when we understand that there is a greater spiritual reality within are we motivated to turn our mind inward. This inner reality or true self can provide us with a true enjoyment, freedom from suffering, and a sublime bliss. This reality can be hinted at in writings, but can be fully known only through experience. One must have a hunger for the inner reality to make the decision to turn the mind inward, or perhaps one must slowly overcome one's prior decision to direct the mind outward.

To be able to turn the mind inward, we must understand how the mind works. In this regard, Swami Prabhavananda and Christopher Isherwood prescribe the following practice. "It is good to spend some time every day simply watching our mind, listening to those drumbeats. We probably shall not like what we see and hear, but we must be very patient and objective. The mind finding itself watched in this way, will gradually grow calmer."[7] In other words, if we learn to watch the mind and understand it, we can catch the attachments and identifications before they spring outward through the senses. As we improve our skill in this respect, the mind becomes more adept at the practice of pratyahara.

Pratyahara leads to mastery of the senses, a unique state. One develops a type of objectivity and a supreme peacefulness, in which sensory experiences do not create feelings of attachment or aversion. We witness without reaction and increasingly mimic the ability of supreme Consciousness to witness.

Beyond this objectivity, the mind becomes more dynamic;

it is one-pointed and free of restless activity. There is a disinclination to seek out sensory experiences—yet we can act in the world without attachment. Because we do not get lost in the morass of sensory experience, we can act with great purpose and effectiveness. When the mental fluctuations come under control, the senses are harnessed. We are able to perceive from a point of balance and to witness without excessive attachment. These abilities allow us to reduce stress. We are not as likely to develop perceptions that set off and maintain the stress response. We have developed a subtle channel for managing stress and promoting our own wellness and effectiveness.

In summary, the yogic concept of sensory functioning is subjective: perceptual experiences are a product of our total physical, mental, and spiritual state. If the mind is attached or disturbed, if the body is out of balance, and if we have no sense of meaning or purpose in life, perception is biased accordingly. These biases can then lead to perception that creates negative emotional patterns and this may lead to an ever-accelerating cycle of stress. In other words, when we are in a state of stress, we are more likely to perceive inner and outer events in a manner that can exacerbate stress. To break the stress cycle it is imperative that we learn the secrets of managing our perceptions. In this regard, the science of yoga has a great deal to offer. The technique of sensory withdrawal, whereby one leads the senses within and experiences a state of peacefulness and quiet, is an essential and often neglected part of stress management. As our perception becomes free, spontaneous, and accurate we are not only more insightful in daily life, but we are also able to further the processes of personality integration and personal growth. We are able to use perception to obtain the feedback and inspiration needed for continuing self-transformation.

CHAPTER 11
Stress, Helplessness, and Hope

John R. Harvey, Ph.D.

Usually when we picture someone experiencing stress we imagine a person who is tense, has too many commitments, and is trying to squeeze too many activities into too little time. We may imagine someone inextricably caught on the treadmill of life, with the internal motor constantly in high gear. We imagine the person to be coping poorly, resorting to caffeine, alcohol, or some other drug to help maintain his frantic pace. This familiar view of stress leads to the image of an individual who eventually simply burns out.

Yet stress is more complex than that; it may be that the person sitting quietly and passively is at just as much risk as the harried individual. It may be that the feelings of being "stuck" in life, of lacking control, and of giving up are equally lethal. Indeed, the person who feels overwhelmed and gives up may be creating a deadly slowdown in the cardiovascular system. The person mourning a loss who feels that life is out of control, may be silently inhibiting his or her immune system and opening the gates

This chapter is adapted from an earlier version, published in Dawn *magazine, Volume 4, Number 2, 1984.*

to pathogens or the growth of cancer.

The giving-up syndrome is the dark, shadowy side of the stress response. Generally it is less understood but is equally as damaging as the hurried and harried approach to life. To fully manage stress we must understand this quieter, less noticeable aspect of the stress response. We must learn to reduce our tendencies toward the giving-up syndrome and use our understanding of this lethal passivity to define a healthy and hardy lifestyle.

Let us consider an example of the giving-up syndrome in a hypothetical laboratory experiment. A white rat moves comfortably in his cage when suddenly from a grid in the floor he receives a painful electric shock. The rat explodes into a flurry of activity, frantically searching for an escape. The shock stops, and slowly the rat's pounding pulse and racing heart slow down. Suddenly another shock comes, and again the rat makes a frantic attempt to escape, but to no avail. The shocks come again and again without predictable interval, pattern, or warning.

Eventually the rat becomes lethargic, stops struggling, and ceases trying to help himself. He gives the appearance of depression and paralysis of the will. When shocked he lies passively with glazed eyes. He loses his ability to learn, for even if some pattern, warning, or escape route is offered, he does not recognize or utilize this information. Important physical changes occur. The heart rate slows, peripheral vascular resistance increases, and cardiac arrhythmias occur. The immune system becomes seriously inhibited, opening the gate to disease, but before any of these diseases can strike, the rat simply crumples and expires.

In this hypothetical experiment the rat becomes helpless and lethargic, and finally dies from giving up. Such results have been found in a number of similar laboratory experiments, and dramatic parallels have been noted with humans. This state or syndrome is usually known as "learned helplessness."[1] In humans it has been described as powerlessness,[2] hopelessness, or the "possum response."[3] This hopelessness/helplessness response may be an integral aspect of stress in general. It has been suggested that helplessness may be a key factor in both cardiac disease[4] and in cancer.[5]

Although humans are not ordinarily subjected to the drastic situation of electric shock, we sometimes see ourselves as assailed by aversive factors—violent crimes, pollution, economic crises, diseases. and wars—that are beyond our control or prediction. Accordingly, depression and the accompanying feelings of hopelessness and helplessness are common mental health problems. For many, a feeling of hope is only a vague and blurry memory from the distant past. Given the significance and prevalence of the giving-up syndrome, it may be useful to study the causes, effects, prevention, and cure of this syndrome.

The Giving-Up Syndrome: Evidence from Animal Research

Some of the most significant work on the syndrome has been done with animals. The results provide the first line of evidence on the existence of a learned state of helplessness and its effects. These results are rich in implications for understanding the giving-up syndrome in humans.

An original, important study in this area was conducted by Martin Seligman and J. Bruce Overmier in 1967,[6] and it involved a startling discovery. Shocks had been delivered to dogs restrained in a harness, and nothing they did could prevent the shock. Subsequently, when these animals were placed in a shuttle box, a device that allows termination of shock by jumping to the other side, a surprising result occurred. When the dogs were shocked in the box, they struggled briefly but after about 30 seconds they lay down passively and accepted the shock; they never learned to escape.

This behavior was labeled "learned helplessness." It was a striking contrast to the behavior of a normal, previously unshocked dog, which would struggle vigorously until it learned to escape shock by jumping to the other side of the box. On successive trials such a dog would become increasingly proficient at escaping shock. Seligman and his colleagues continued this work with further studies using dogs, fish, cats, and rats, with the same basic results. Based upon these data a theory regarding learned helplessness was developed. The key aspect of the theory is that uncontrollable aversive events lead to significant changes in an organism's emotions, behavior, and physiology. It was theorized that the organism develops an expectation that outcome is independent of response. The specific effects of learned helplessness are described as follows:

1. Decreased Motivation—Helpless animals were less likely to initiate any voluntary response that might help them adjust.

2. Cognitive Disruption—An animal that has "given up" seems to have difficulty perceiving things that might be helpful or useful, such as an escape route.

3. Emotional Disturbance—The initial response to uncontrollable stimuli is one of heightened fear and high arousal. However, as the animal increasingly confronts uncontrollable factors, this arousal turns into passivity, inhibition, and depression.

Seligman emphasizes that it is the lack of control of aversive events that seems to create a belief that outcome is entirely independent of the response, that there is not value or use in responding. Learned helplessness may be a temporary effect, and after a time more energetic behavior may return. However, the longer and more intense the period of lack of control, the longer the helplessness will persist.

Other researchers in the field believe that lack of

control of aversive events is not the only significant factor in the appearance of learned helplessness; they believe that lack of predictability is an equally important dimension.[7] Unpredictable aversive events are significantly more stressful than predictable aversive events. For example, in a study in which two groups of rats received the same number of shocks, the animals that received a warning light prior to every onset of shock showed considerably less stomach ulceration.

Additional analysis of so-called experimental neurosis research has underlined the importance of predictability. In these studies the animal typically is taught that one signal (for example, the figure of a circle) means food, while another signal (such as an ellipse) indicates that no food or even a shock will be forthcoming. The signals serve to predict these significant events.

When these signals are altered to the point that the animal can no longer make a clear discrimination (for example, the circle and ellipse change shape and come to approximate each other), remarkable changes occur in the animals. First they become highly agitated and aggressive, and then they progress to a state of lethargy and depression, a state recognizable as learned helplessness. As researchers, Susan Mineka and John Kihlstrom note, "unpredictable events have profound emotional, somatic and cognitive effects on the organism."[8]

Helplessness can also result in sudden death. In a well-known experiment, C.P. Richter took wild rats, which are known for their stamina and resourcefulness, and held them until they stopped struggling.[9] Then he clipped their whiskers, a crucial sense organ. When these animals were placed in a vat of water, they would swim in an agitated fashion for several minutes and then suddenly sink beneath the surface. In sharp contrast, other rats that had been held and released before they ceased to struggle, thereby learning that escape was possible, would swim for as long as sixty hours before they slipped beneath the water.

An even more striking finding from this study was that the rats that gave up quickly died in a most unusual manner. In the typical situation of sudden death the heart speeds up due to activation of the sympathetic branch of the autonomic nervous system. However, each of these rats died as a result of the heart's slowing down (bradycardia). Autopsy revealed that the heart was engorged with blood, showing that a parasympathetic death, a death of relaxation or giving up, had occurred.

When Richter injected atropine (a substance that blocks parasympathetic discharge) prior to the experiment, these pretreated rats showed significantly less mortality. The conclusion reached by Richter was that the rats that drowned quickly had simply given up the struggle.

Several experiments by Seligman and his co-workers have verified this phenomenon of death by giving up. In these experiments rats were exposed to inescapable shock. The intent was to subsequently place the animals in water and determine how long they would survive compared with animals that had received escapable shock. However, many of the rats receiving the inescapable shock died while receiving the shocks: "To our surprise six of the twelve lay down, paws splayed beneath the grids, and died in the box during mild, long-duration shocks. Their hearts were engorged with blood."[10]

A related phenomenon is the catatonic response that some animals display when they are overwhelmed by a predator. For example, when a rodent is seized by a hawk it may freeze, and even if dropped may remain motionless and unresponsive for a number of minutes before getting up and scampering away. Laboratory research by M.A. Hofer found that rodents exposed to a sudden loud noise, to the silhouette of a hawk, or to a snake showed this response for as long as thirty minutes.[11] Analysis of their cardiac response showed the telltale, dramatic slowing of the heart rate. In some instances subtle arrhythmias were apparent. These rodents were also subsequently found to be more susceptible to sudden death from other causes. In other words, their giving up, or "possum response," had made them more vulnerable to other stressors.

Application of inescapable shock appears to create an even greater vulnerability. Chickens that had received inescapable shock and were then exposed to a predator remained immobile five times longer than normal chickens, and some even died during the immobilization.[12]

Remarkable findings on sudden death have also been noted with primates. Here the precursor seems to be a type of grief response that is analogous to what humans may experience. For instance, it has been observed that if a primate is suddenly separated from a parent or if a primate's parent or mate dies, the animal may lapse into the progression of a short period of agitation followed by lethargy and depression, concluding in a death that cannot be traced to any definite pathogen. Seligman quotes a particularly poignant description from the work of the famous anthropologist Jane Goodall. The passage concerns the death of Flo, a chimpanzee, and the subsequent fate of her son, Flint.

Flo lay down on a rock, toward the side of a stream and simply expired. She was quite old. Flint stayed near her corpse. He grabbed one of her arms and tried to pull her up by the hand. The night of her death he slept close to the body, and by the following morning, he showed signs of extreme depression.

After that, no matter where he might wander off to, he kept returning to his mother's body. It was the maggots which, at last, drove him away; he'd try to shake the maggots off her and they would swarm on him.

Finally he stopped coming back. But he did remain in the area comprising about 50 square yards; and he wouldn't move any further away from the place where Flo had died. And in 10 days he had lost about a third of his body weight. He also developed a strange, glazed look.

At last Flint died too; he died very close to the spot where his mother had died. In fact, the day before he had returned to sit on the very rock where Flo had lain down (by then we had removed her body and buried her).

The results of the postmortem have been negative. They indicated that although he had a certain parasite load and one or two bugs, there was nothing sufficient in itself to cause death. And so the major cause of death had to be grief.[13]

While the research reviewed above points to parasympathetically induced bradycardia and arrhythmias as the physiological mechanisms leading to death, some recent research points to another mechanism that must be given consideration: the inhibition of the immune system. Research by Steven Meier and his colleagues[14] has investigated the effects of controllable and uncontrollable stressors on the immune system functioning of rats. Four groups of rats received either controllable electric shock they could turn off, the same amount of uncontrollable shock, exposure to the apparatus with no shock, or no change at all. The researchers measured the proliferation of immune system T-cells in response to a simulated invasion of foreign cells. The rats exposed to controllable stress showed T-cell proliferation, indicating a strong immune system response like the unstressed group, whereas rats exposed to uncontrollable stress showed a significant suppression of T-cell production, indicating a suppression of immune function. Similar results have been found in studying young monkeys separated from their mothers. There is also direct evidence that lowered lymphocyte production can occur in humans after the loss of a spouse.

Meier and his colleagues have also looked at the effects of stress on the so-called NK, or "natural killer," cells. These NK cells play a particularly important role in immune system function, as they search for and destroy tumors. They apparently patrol the body and effectively reduce the probability of cancer. As might be expected, rats exposed to uncontrollable stressors showed lower levels of NK cells. Meier and his colleagues note other research indicating that humans who react to high levels of life change with anxiety and depression are more likely to show lower NK cell activity. Women who passively accept breast cancer have lower levels of NK activity than those who show anger and a more active fighting mode.

The key point emphasized by Meier and his colleagues is that a belief that one has control profoundly influences the psychological and physiological response to negative events. Individuals who feel that events are out of control, who have no hope for change, who have given up, and who are consequently anxious and depressed are most likely to develop a host of physical symptoms, including the potentially deadly suppression of the immune system.

In summary, the existence of a giving-up or learned helplessness syndrome has been clearly substantiated in animal research. It is caused by the presentation of unpredictable aversive events over which the animal has no control. The effects of the syndrome can be summarized as follows:

1. Behavioral changes, including decreased motivation to respond and decreased cognitive skills in learning new control-relevant information. The effects seem to guarantee that the helpless animal will remain helpless.

2. Emotional changes, typically involving initial agitation followed by depression and lethargy.

3. Physiological changes, which in the most dramatic cases can lead to sudden death. Excessive parasympathetic discharge and immune system suppression appear to be the

major pathways for these physiological changes.

These changes and effects must be seen, however, in the context of helplessness as a cumulative state. The more frequent and intense the experience of uncontrollable and unpredictable events, the more vulnerable the organism becomes to dramatic negative effects. On the other hand, organisms that are given time to recover seem to bounce back rather nicely. Recovery is speeded by previous experiences of recovery. Also, the opportunity to be active and competent on one's own behalf seems to lessen the impact of aversive events. With this picture of the giving-up syndrome in mind, it now becomes important to examine the next line of evidence: the giving-up syndrome in humans.

The Giving-Up Syndrome in Humans

A number of studies with human subjects also have demonstrated the cognitive, behavioral, and motivational effects of helplessness. One issue in these studies has been the effect of a sense of control. For instance, one study showed that when subjects can control the intensity of shocks they receive, they report less discomfort than when the same degree of shocks are administered without control.[15] In another study, two groups of subjects listened to loud random noise.[16] One group could control the noise, and showed better frustration tolerance, committed fewer errors on a performance test, and even rated the noise as less aversive than the group without control over the noise.

In a study with female subjects, those who could advance travel slides according to their own preference were better able to tolerate having one hand immersed in ice water than a group for whom the slides were automatically advanced, and still better than a group that had no diverting slides.[17] The implications of these studies are that control of any kind—whether it is direct control over the noxious stimuli or of some other factor—increases tolerance for aversive stimuli, while the lack of control in the face of aversive stimuli leads to decrements in performance levels and greater subjective feelings of distress.

In a study with humans that resembled learned helplessness studies done with animals, subjects who had no control of shocks and no way to predict them were found to be less likely to learn control in a subsequent phase of the experiment in which control was possible.[18] The experience of lack of control and unpredictability seemed to make the subsequent learning of control more difficult. Again, a key aspect of learned helplessness appears to be the subject's belief that outcome and response are independent of one another. We can expect, then, to see the same types of results with learned helplessness in humans as in animals. These are (1) a lowered rate of initiating voluntary responses, (2) a negative cognitive set, (3) a reduction in aggression, (4) loss of appetite, and (5) physiological changes.

As interesting as these laboratory findings are, the most dramatic work on the effects of helplessness in humans comes from clinical work. One of the foremost authorities in this area is Lawrence LeShan, who has conducted extensive psychotherapy with terminal cancer patients and has carefully studied the link between emotional factors and cancer. One manner in which LeShan has substantiated this connection is through the study of cancer mortality data. He analyzed the data on women who died of cancer during the years 1929-31. His conclusion was that cancer deaths were most common for widows and least common for single individuals, across all ages. Further review of these data revealed that married individuals with a greater probability of meaningful relationships (that is, married individuals with children) had a low incidence of cancer. Taken together, the findings indicate that, in LeShan's words, "any situation that tends to disrupt the formation of strong meaningful relationships can be predicted to result in higher cancer mortality rates."[19]

LeShan also did extensive interviews, psychological tests, and psychotherapy with other cancer patients. Analyzing his clinical data, he noted two factors that distinguished cancer patients from non-cancer controls. These were (1) loss of reason for existence, and (2) an inability to express anger and resentment. It is important to note that the first factor, a loss of meaning in life, typically arose when the individual lost a significant person, usually a spouse. Often the individual seemed to depend entirely on a central relationship, the loss of which was catastrophic and threw the individual into a state of utter despair. In terms of the second factor, an inability to express anger and resentment, LeShan determined that cancer patients often presented a facade of affability and goodness while repressing aggressive and hostile feelings.

The syndrome that LeShan identified is clearly a type of helplessness; the individual feels isolated and cut off from others, alienated from himself, unable to aggressively defend himself, and without hope for the future. LeShan speculates that the person who feels helpless inhibits immune function, which in turn allows the aberrant cancer cells to flourish. The immune system suppression may be linked to hormones, which in turn are definitely affected by emotional factors. It would seem that the giving-up syndrome opens the gates to cancer.

The clinical work of O. C. Simonton points to similar conclusions on the relationship between emotions and cancer.[20] He found that the onset of cancer is often preceded by a cluster of stressful events with which the individual feels incapable of dealing. In this situation the individual is likely to see no solution and no escape unless it is via the avenue of death. Such people see themselves as powerless in the face of their cancer. Simonton also hypothesizes that emotionally-based immune system suppression is the mechanism linking despair to cancer.

The physical effects of helplessness may be even more dramatic in the case of sudden death in humans. The study of phenomena such as voodoo deaths suggests that when an individual perceives events as being out of control, parasympathetic activation takes over. This involves a slowing of the heart rate. As the bradycardia proceeds, the chance of severe arrhythmias arises, and death may follow.[21] In some instances there may be a rapid alternation between activation and inhibition—the cardiovascular system literally goes out of control in the face of overwhelming conflict.

The extreme examples of cancer and heart failure illustrate the dramatic and deadly effects of helplessness in many life situations, yet the onset of physical illness leading eventually to death may be slower and more complex. A compelling example is the case of Kennedy Space Center workers during the mid-to-late sixties. These highly trained and achievement-oriented individuals were caught in a huge and overwhelming conflict. On the one hand there was tremendous pressure for achievement, high visibility, and complex work demands. On the other hand, it was clear there would be budget cuts and layoffs. "In short, the project demanded an ever increasing if not frenzied pace of production with the ultimate reward of nearly inevitable dismissal, financial loss and loss of professional identity."[22]

These workers displayed a divorce rate of 75%, a high incidence of neuroticism, anxiety, and despair, and a nation-leading per capita consumption of alcohol. They also displayed a rate of sudden death 50% higher than the general population. Certainly the arousal and job demands placed stress on these individuals; however, it seems that the feeling of hopelessness made the situation lethal.

There are other reports that illustrate how giving up and helplessness can lead to death. W.B. Cannon, for instance, has reviewed examples of sudden death in primitive cultures. He cites examples from Brazil, Africa, New Zealand, and Australia in which individuals who were cursed died within a day. He provides the following dramatic description of a typical individual's response to being "boned" (that is, cursed) by a witch doctor:

> He stands aghast with his eyes staring at the treacherous pointer, and with his hands lifted to ward off the lethal medium, which he imagines is pouring into his body. His cheeks blanch, and his eyes become glassy, and the expression of his face becomes horribly distorted. He attempts to shriek but usually the sound chokes in his throat, and all that one might see is froth at his mouth. His body begins to twitch involuntarily. He sways backward and falls to the ground, and after a short time appears to be in a swoon. He finally composes himself, goes to his hut and there frets to death.[23]

A South African physician named Burrell reports witnessing six instances in which middle-aged Bantu men were cursed that they would die before sunset—and in fact they all did.[24] In each of these cases the autopsy did not provide any information regarding the cause of death. In reviewing these accounts, Martin Seligman states that the crucial element is the individual's belief that he is utterly helpless in the face of a pronouncement of doom.[25] Accordingly he shows passivity, depression, submission, and finally death.

In Western society, although there are no clearly recognized witch doctors and hexes, there are, nevertheless, frequent instances of sudden death. Researchers who carefully examined 170 instances of sudden death found specific categories of incidents that preceded demise.[26] Prominent among them are (1) the death of a loved one, (2) acute grief, (3) threatened loss of a loved one, (4) mourning or anniversary of mourning, and (5) dramatic loss of status and self-esteem. These situations appear to create in some people a sense that things are irrevocably out of control and a feeling of hopelessness and helplessness.

Institutional settings may also provide a context within which helplessness and inexplicable sudden death may occur.[27] In such settings, in which control and predictability are low, it is easy for patients to give up. Prisoners of war who are stripped of their identities and of their accustomed functioning, and who believe they have no hope may give up mentally, become glassy-eyed and passive, and die in the same environmental circumstances in which other prisoners cling to hope, exert their will and survive.

Nursing home patients are another group that may be quite vulnerable to death from helplessness. In this regard N.A. Ferrari studied seventy-five elderly patients admitted to a nursing home.[28] Seventeen of the patients were convinced that they had no choice as to whether or not to enter the nursing home. Eight of them died within four weeks, and sixteen were dead within ten weeks. In striking contrast, of the thirty-eight patients who considered several placement options but chose the nursing home, only one had died after ten weeks. Thus it appears that loss of choice and control can bring forth the helplessness syndrome and ensuing death.

Furthermore, it seems that the elderly are quite sensitive to changes in the routine and structure of their lives. In a situation where a geriatric ward burned and patients had to be moved while repairs were made, the subtle vestiges of control and predictability were apparently swept away: the death rate jumped from 7.5% to 20% within four weeks.[29]

The subtle inner science of yoga may provide another perspective on the manner in which negative emotions influence physiology. According to yoga science, human beings consist of various levels of being, called sheaths.[30] The outermost and grossest, or most material, sheath is the body. Within the body sheath, and more subtle than it, is an energy level or pranic sheath. This subtle level of energy maintains the body, yet is itself maintained by a further level, the mind. Thus, the mental body, the finest of the three sheaths, maintains the energy body, which in turn maintains the physical body.

Hopelessness leads to a decrease and withdrawal of mental energy. This, in turn, leads to a decrease in the energy body or pranic field. The body field is no longer correctly maintained as these finer and supporting fields are weakened. Hence the natural processes of decay are accelerated, and disease may readily occur.

Often this phenomenon is quite specific. A physician who practices holistic medicine related a case of a woman with significant degenerative eye disease who said that she couldn't bear to look at things and that she saw no hope in her life. Here it would appear that the physical malady was preceded by a definite and specific mental disruption—and a subsequent organ-specific disruption of the energy field.

Although the yogic concept of a mediating energy field may be difficult to grasp for those of us raised in a culture that believes in a mind-body dichotomy, it may be worthwhile to attempt to appreciate this integrative perspective of layers or sheaths. In fact, the notion of an energy field provides us with the best understanding of how the mind influences the body.

Actually the influences are even more profound than those of conscious mental functioning. Yoga science states that there are also two more levels or sheaths that support the mind-energy-body complex. The first of these is the wisdom sheath, which deals with the experience of a higher mind, with intuition, and with awareness of the unconscious. And finally there is a blissful sheath that deals with transcendental consciousness. These last two levels are part of what might be called the subtle body, and it follows that disruptions such as a lack of meaning in life and lack of a spiritual perspective may create subsequent imbalances in the mind-energy-body complex.

The Origins of Hopelessness

LeShan and Simonton have both noted that a certain type of personality or world view seems to be most vulnerable to cancer. This view appears to develop early in life. The first factor identified is an unresponsive childhood in which the full spectrum of nurturing experiences is not provided. The child experiences a sense of isolation and may come to believe that intense and meaningful relationships are dangerous and can bring pain. Often there is an abbreviated childhood. He or she may be prematurely cast into a role with responsibility due to the death of a family member or the birth of an immediately following sibling. Dependency needs are often unmet. The child is unable to express emotional energy in the context of relationships; the child's vital energy is often bottled up.

Also the child may develop a number of negative habits of thinking and typically misinterpret the actions of others and the demands of the environment; the child sees criticism and rejection where there is none. Another pattern is black and white thinking, in which one characterizes oneself or others as either totally good or totally bad. Such cognitive patterns have been labeled "schemas" by Aaron Beck and his co-workers, and have been found to be the means by which depressed people maintain their depression.[31] Moreover, these patterns or schemas organize one's conscious experience and result in what Beck has labeled the "cognitive triad" of negative view of self, negative view of ongoing experiences, and negative view of the future.

In addition to this depressive tendency, individuals who are vulnerable to helplessness often grow up with a mechanistic view of the world. They feel that fate weaves an inexorable course. They believe that good things in life can come only from extremely hard work. These individuals doubt their ability to produce and feel that they are unworthy of good things. They are also often emotionally blocked, and are unable to express their strong, real emotions.

These early experiences, beliefs, and thought patterns constitute what LeShan describes as phase one in the development of hopelessness. Phase two consists of the individual's discovery and development either of a meaningful relationship with another person or significant satisfaction from work activities. The person experiences a sense of acceptance, competence, and relative contentment with life. However, the fall comes during phase three, in which the meaningful relationship or satisfying work role is lost. Utter despair arises, a despair that exceeds any of the phase-one unhappiness. The person believes that life holds no hope. Cancer may then develop within a year.

LeShan has found that phase-three people hold a uniquely negative view of themselves and the world. They assume that:

1. Objects and people outside themselves can't bring help.

2. There is no possibility of development or change. Things will remain bad.

3. No action can ease the loneliness and hurt. All attempts only serve to validate this point.

Interestingly enough, phase-three individuals usually continue to function, and may on the surface appear placid and even hard-working. But they live without hope. They feel trapped, and in the face of this inner predicament death stands as an acceptable escape. Cancer is seen as one more piece of evidence that life is indeed hopeless.

LeShan describes Jenny, who was dying of cancer: "In her quiet voice Jenny told me that she was not surprised at this outcome to her life. She had always felt that nothing would ever go right for her, that she had no real hope of happiness."[32] The experience of despair is even more dramatically portrayed in a quote from another cancer patient: "You know how it is with a house with no insulation and with cracks in the walls. The more you put in heat, the more it leaks out. You can never get warm. I always knew that's how it was with me in life. I had to keep putting out, and there was never any reflection back at me. If I was going to get warm inside, I'd have to do it alone, and no matter how much you do, you can't do that."[33]

Simonton points to a similar developmental pattern. He believes that there are five phases in psychological development that make an individual vulnerable to cancer. The first involves a decision in childhood to incorporate rigid rules about what kind of person one will or will not be. For example, a child might decide that he will never display anger. Secondly, the individual experiences a high number of stressful life events, such as the death of a spouse, role changes, or retirement.

Thirdly, these stressors leave the individual in a problem situation that he does not know how to solve. This means that his rules don't allow him to cope with the situation. Fourthly, as the conviction grows that the problem can't be solved, a feeling of being trapped and helpless pervades the individual. Finally the individual gives up; as Simonton notes, the person is simply "running in place,"[34] with no real sense of vitality and meaning in life. This constellation of factors seems to exist in many of Simonton's patients.

In contrast to this lifelong psychosocial development that can lead to cancer, other researchers have examined helplessness in a more immediate time context and with other physiological and behavioral consequences. The precursors of this type of helplessness are a series of uncontrollable and unpredictable life changes. Typical changes include the death of a spouse or other family member, loss of status, extreme physical threat, hospitalization, relocation, retirement, being assigned a social level connoting inferiority, engaging in work that is perceived as demeaning, losing physical independence, and experiencing chronic physical pain.

With such stressors in mind, J.F. Miller has suggested

a nine-stage progression in the development of hopelessness in which a person increasingly fails to reach goals to solve problems, or even to come up with possible solutions, and consequently loses faith in self and others, finally giving up.[35] This progression toward hopelessness is accelerated by coping behaviors that use avoidance. Most significant among these is the pattern of denial of reality, the suppression and repression of emotions, and the tendency to minimize.

With these avoidance behaviors operative, the person typically interprets the stressors he encounters as evidence of a tragic and inexorable fate. Social withdrawal and the termination of formerly satisfying activities occurs. The individual passively accepts things. Sleep and appetite become disturbed, thereby draining the individual of physical energy. Making decisions becomes harder. The individual may turn to drugs and alcohol for solace and relief. Within the context of these behaviors the web of helplessness grows.

G. L. Engel describes this as the "giving up-given up complex."[36] He notes five characteristics of this experience: (1) feeling that one is at the end of one's rope, at an impasse, (2) having a poor self-image and feeling incompetent and out of control, (3) having a loss of gratification from roles and relationships, (4) feeling that there is no continuity between past, present, and future, and (5) recalling memories of previous helpless states.

Helplessness may also be considered as a spiritual impasse in which an individual loses faith and no longer perceives any meaning in life or any hope for self-expression. Tarthang Tulku Rinpoche, a Tibetan Buddhist teacher, describes a special kind of spiritual despair that can arise when we block our instrinsic flow of growth and change: "We do not wish to make the effort to change, but fighting change takes an even greater effort. Trying to prevent change in our lives is like trying to swim against the current of a flowing river. This way of being exhausts and frustrates us until a defeated quality begins to permeate our lives."[37]

Obviously the giving-up syndrome arises from a constellation of factors: certain experiences in early family life, childhood, and adolescence can influence us to adopt emotional and cognitive habits and beliefs that make us more vulnerable to feelings of helplessness. Exposure to multiple uncontrollable and unpredictable negative events sets the immediate stage for hopelessness. Our inability to grow drives the sense of despair to the deepest levels of our being. Then our coping behaviors determine how severe the hopelessness will be, how long it will last, and how profound the effects will be in terms of our behavior, thoughts, emotions, and physical health.

Recovering Hope

Just as there is a constellation of factors that leads to hopelessness and giving up, there are, fortunately, a number of factors that lead one to establish, maintain, and strengthen a sense of hope. Heretofore we have described the condition of hopelessness; now we must consider hope itself.

A beginning may be to reverse the definition of hopelessness. A person with hope believes that there is a relationship between what he does and what happens. It is an expectation greater than zero that a goal, need, or desire will be met. Moreover, the individual with hope believes that he has something to do with reaching that goal, need, or desire. But hope is deeper than an expectation or a probability. It is a type of faith. J.F. Miller has described hope as "the affect that accompanies faith."[38]

The level and depth of hope depend on our expectations and goals. The individual whose hopes center on material goods can quickly readjust if his goals are not met, and still maintain his hope. On the other hand, a deeper set of goals concerning relationships, accomplishments, and self-improvement demands a greater investment of psychic energy, and consequently loss here is deeper and more profound.

Yet the deepest level of hope concerns the very meaning of life and reason for existence. Sometimes in the throes of discouragement we are forced to develop a deep sense of hope and faith. For example, while in the seemingly hopeless situation of a concentration camp, the noted existentialist Viktor Frankl rose above the immediate suffering by picturing himself in a warm and pleasant lecture hall speaking to an attentive audience on the psychology of the concentration camp. This allowed him to not only objectify and thereby lessen his present suffering, but gave him a vision for the future and an immediate task—to begin preparing for those future lectures. Such an outlook was crucial for survival. As Frankl writes, "The prisoner who had lost faith in the future—his future—was doomed. With his loss of belief in the future, he also lost his spiritual hold; he let himself decline and become subject to mental and physical decay."[39]

Just as hopelessness weakens our energy to respond, creates a negative cognitive set, and inhibits our learning of control-relevant information, hope has the opposite effect. With hope, we always have more to draw on in our energy reservoir; hope is profoundly energizing. With hope, we tend to interpret circumstances as providing confirmation or substantiation of our faith. With hope, we are alert to ideas and skills that can bring us to our dreams and goals.

We have noted that giving up has profound negative effects on our health. Conversely, a state of hope and a sense of meaning have beneficial effects on our body. With hope, the healing process is accelerated. In this connection, LeShan notes: "It is the individual who, accepting his own being as valid, continually seeks self-fulfillment—the individual whose hopes for his own full rich life are sufficiently high to enable him to deal with temporary setbacks—who appears most resistant to cancer."[40]

Finally, in our effort to define hope it may be interesting to look at the dictionary definitions. Webster's New Twentieth Century Unabridged Dictionary defines hope as "a desire for some good, accompanied with at least a slight expectation of obtaining it, or a belief that it is obtainable," "confidence in a future event; the highest degree of well-founded expectations of good," and a now archaic usage as "trust; reliance." Perhaps there is something special and essential about that last archaic definition. Perhaps the essence of hope is a feeling of trust in life, a feeling and belief that one can rely on the world around him for nourishment and sustenance.

We have noted that the experience of hopelessness stems from our perception of events around us. Giving up is a function of both the conscious and the unconscious mind. Accordingly, to recover or vitalize hope we must determine what can be done in terms of working with the various levels of the mind.

The first approach to vitalizing hope is directed toward the conscious mind and involves gaining information. People benefit by understanding all aspects of a stressful life event. Knowledge makes things more understandable and thereby more bearable. It is interesting to look at the results of a study of fifty-six individuals undergoing therapy for chronic illness.[41] The strategy employed most frequently by these individuals was information seeking. This involved focusing on details of care, learning about illness-required changes in habits and diet, questioning the rationale for therapy, and comparing staff responses to the same questions.

Of course, stressful events such as the death of a loved one often appear to defy understanding. In spite of this, there is information to be gained. We can learn about the circumstances of the loved one's death. We can attempt to probe this mystery of death by reading about death, discussing it with others, and attempting to see death in a broader perspective. We can look to the great philosophical and religious traditions and see how they explain death. This does not mean that we will not feel sad or that we will not miss our loved one. It does mean that we will have some understanding of the event, and with that knowledge, hopelessness declines. The event may, with sufficient knowledge, be seen as an event in a greater system.

A second approach to recovering hope involves rational thinking. As we have noted, individuals who have given up often have erroneous and biased ways of interpreting information. One of the first changes is to challenge all assumptions. For example, if a person believes that he will never find satisfaction or meaningful love again, this must first be seen as an assumption, not a fact. The person may then challenge the belief by questioning: "How do I know I won't find love again? What is the evidence that I can't find satisfaction?" By such inner dialogue and self-analysis the person can weaken the rigid, negative cognitive set and begin to appraise the situation differently. We must keep in mind that our rules and assumptions make us vulnerable to the perception of uncontrollability and unpredictability.

Aaron Beck, who has extensively studied the logic of depressed and discouraged people, has found a number of types of erroneous and faulty thinking.[42] These include overgeneralizing, rigid black and white thinking, overpersonalizing events, focusing on fragments of evidence instead of the whole picture, and magnifying or minimizing crucial data. In the system of cognitive therapy that Beck has devised, the therapist forms an alliance with the client and together they work on evaluating the client's cognitive habits and developing more objective and logical habits of thinking. Numerous studies have shown that this is a highly effective method for overcoming despair.

Miller utilizes the term "reality surveillance" as a cognitive method for maintaining hope.[43] Reality surveillance and reasoned thinking bring about rationalization and readjustment of goals. This can actually be a means to strengthen the will. The helpless-hopeless individual typically dwells on distant, unrealistic goals. But if more immediate goals are set and the individual can reach these, the will is strengthened. We might, for instance, pledge to ourselves to keep our room clean for a week, to exercise daily, or to cut back on junk food for five days.

As such goals are reached, our will becomes creative and strong. A feedback loop is created whereby we begin to see ourselves as people who "can do." Thus, will and hope can strengthen and reinforce each other.

As this process continues, we eventually see that control and prediction come from inside ourselves. This revolution in perspective takes place in two stages. First we begin to evaluate external experiences in a more objective manner. Then we become less dependent on external factors and experience a heightened sense of control and an awareness that what happens outside has its origins within ourselves.

Self-analysis brings us to the third approach to recovering hope, which is self-confrontation and self-acceptance. In fact, LeShan sees this stage of facing ourselves as crucial if there is to be any hope of reversing the process of concern. The key question for us to address is: What do we really want? Answering this question can be difficult, for we frequently deny, devalue, or cover with shame certain vital aspects of ourselves.

In such cases there is an embryonic self within that must be delivered. Profound unhappiness, discontent, self-hatred, and repression are the labor pains accompanying this birth. As LeShan notes, "Unhappiness almost invariably indicates the existence of a road not taken, a talent undeveloped, a self not recognized."[44]

Actually, the process of self-confrontation often brings forth a number of questions, such as: What do I really want? What gives me a sense of meaning? What do I find worth doing? Do I absolutely have to have love? As such questions are answered, the person gradually becomes able to answer the question: What is the first step to take in realizing my goals?

This entails delineating action, and action implies reactivation of the will and hope. The oft-repeated observation that the journey of a thousand miles begins with a single step is applicable here. In recovering hope, the individual must see the goal and take the first step. Hope arises from doing, acting, and reaching. One cannot just think things over and have hope, but must begin to take steps toward the goal.

LeShan cautions that the stage of confrontation is not easy and may bring in the classic existential crisis. A number of avoidance habits may interfere. The tendency to minimize, repress, and deny obstructs the process of self-confrontation. It may be a struggle to come to grips with oneself. Hence a period of solitude may prove to be quite useful in the process of self-confrontation. Often, too, a supportive relationship can help provide the crucial momentum to penetrate self-imposed restraints.

A result of self-confrontation is a healthy self-acceptance; the individual incorporates his true desires and accepts himself. LeShan calls this the third road. Most of his patients originally saw only two roads available to them on the journey of life. One was to be the way others wanted them to be and to be miserable inside but at least accepted. The second road was to be the way they wanted to be, but be rejected. With this no-win outlook, they felt trapped and hopeless.

But with self-confrontation and self-acceptance, one achieves self-integration. As one gracefully expresses his true self, others will accept him as well. Much of the rejection we perceive is our own self-hatred projected outward. The criticism of others may also be necessary in order for us to learn to become resistant to negative suggestions and to deal with criticism in a healthy and constructive manner.

Often our true self may be imploring us to overcome our self-centeredness and to work for the benefit of others. Such an orientation can give a richer and more satisfying sense of meaning to life. In fact the therapeutic effect of caring for other beings—plants and animals, as well as people—is well known.

LeShan notes that to truly accept oneself, one must acknowledge past self-rejection and rejection by others. Age-regression, free association, intensive interviewing, and recalling prior instances of successful self-integration may be ways to accomplish this. He also notes that novels, poems, and movies may help this process of integration. Patients dealing with catastrophic illness are frequently open to the meanings of artistic creations that deal with despair and loss of the self.

An excerpt from LeShan may help the reader to better understand self-hatred and the development of self-acceptance. LeShan relates the following experience of employing an age-regression technique with a patient named Stuart:

> Stuart remembered lying alone, feeling terribly sad. Because of his father's rejection, Stuart said he had felt that "I must have done something terrible." But he could not imagine what it was: "I guess I felt that it was just being me that was so terrible."
>
> I asked Stuart what he would feel like doing, opening the door and looking in on himself, as the child he had been gazed up expectantly from the bed. He replied: "Going out and closing the door behind me, I guess. There's nothing to say to him at all."

Some forty hours of therapy later, the same scene was visualized once again. Asked the same question—what he would feel like doing on opening the door—Stuart looked at me indignantly and said: "Take him in my arms and hug him, of course. What else would you do with a poor kid like that?"[45]

A fourth approach to facilitating hope is a paradigm shift, or a radically different view of the world. As previously noted, those who are predisposed to hopelessness often are heavily invested in a materialistic cause-and-effect view of the world. The work of self-analysis, self-confrontation, and self-acceptance typically opens the person to appreciate a new way of considering his experiences.

The first level of this shift is to what might be viewed as a humanistic paradigm. Here the very fact of existence is seen as a positive state. The opportunity to learn and grow emotionally is a blessing of life.

From this paradigm every experience has its positive, growth-producing aspects. So-called life stressors can be reframed as opportunities for growth. Even the smallest experience can be richly appreciated. Miller calls this "maximizing the experience."[46] Each event of the day can be savored—the taste and aroma of tea, the tartness of a grapefruit, the warmth of the sun, the color of the sky.

In the tradition of meditation and more recently in the Gestalt therapy movement, this experience is called "being in the now." One lets go of worries about the past and projections of the future and unfolds in the present. When one is in the now a positive, healthful, emotional state unfolds.

One may also see things entirely within a spiritual paradigm. In this outlook, whatever occurs in life is viewed as part of the process of spiritual unfoldment. All life is a manifestation of a supreme eternal Consciousness.[47] The true self within is a source of joy and bliss and unending hope. As one becomes absorbed in this paradigm, hopelessness becomes impossible. It is seen to be a mirage built upon a false view of reality. With knowledge of one's true Self, creative will is activated. It is interesting to note that immersion in spirituality is also one of the most utilized strategies of individuals who cope with life stressors. In fact, it is often the duress of life that forces us to look within and see the reality of our nature. Many experience this spiritual awakening by feeling the totality and power of God's infinite love.

All of these approaches to recovering hope may be facilitated by the process of meditation. Meditation is a resting of the mind so that we can look clearly and accurately at the world. Meditation strengthens our ability to watch the erroneous thoughts in the mind and to avoid becoming swept away by them. We learn that if we let go of locked-in, repetitive thought patterns, we often easily find the solution to a problem. We learn a creative process of inner listening.

But more importantly, meditation is an ongoing process of self-integration and self-discovery. By means of meditation, we quiet the mind and begin to seek our true self. On this journey many of the harsh memories and repressed emotions, the limiting factors of mind, may float to the surface of awareness, where we can acknowledge them and sweep them away. In this manner the mind is purified and we move toward greater acceptance of our self and a greater appreciation of the opportunities and pleasures that life provides. The practice of meditation enables us to take the energy from negative patterns and transform it into positive growth.

Once we have revitalized our sense of hope, we can begin to adapt to whatever problem, illness, or loss is troubling us. That is to say, we can continue with purpose, hope, and direction in life. We become able to acknowledge the illness or loss and transcend it through self-acceptance, hope, and constructive action.

Although we have focused on the mental and spiritual aspects of recovering hope, it would be unwise to ignore the dimensions of body and energy. Just as the body is affected by hopelessness, so also, conversely, the state of the body can influence our level of hope. Patterns of sound nutrition create a healthy biochemical field in which the internal chemistry of hope may flourish. Also, the strength and endurance acquired from exercise may transfer to our mind the strength and endurance we need to cope with significant life stressors. In fact, it seems that habits of good self-care can be a cushion when we are confronted with a hopeless situation. By maintaining a daily practice of beneficial exercising during a crisis, we are starting the process of rebuilding.

In the tradition of yoga, energy is intimately related with the breath. The giving-up response is linked to exaggerated and elongated exhalation, the well-known sigh of depression. This breathing pattern saps the vital energy for both the mind and body. Addressing this energy imbalance is vitally important. Activities such as jogging, swimming, and other aerobic exercises force us to inhale, to breathe in very deeply, and such exercises have been linked to overcoming depression and inspiring a more hopeful outlook. Breath awareness and breathing exercises emphasizing balance between inhalation and exhalation can also be useful. Breathing techniques, exercise programs, and dietary wisdom are explained earlier in this book. These are important channels to facilitate hope. Thus, there are many ways to restore hope and reactivate our creative will. The effort to restore hope is worth it. In the words of David Hume: "A propensity to hope and joy is real riches; one to fear and sorrow, real poverty."

CHAPTER 12
Chakras and the Origins of Stress

Swami Ajaya, Ph.D.

As long as one is absorbed in and identified with the phenomenal reality, the world of names and forms, he is bound to experience stress; he cannot avoid it. To imagine that one can enjoy a stress-free existence in such a state is pure fantasy. This must be so, because phenomenal existence is established by way of stress. Stress is its very nature. The unitary consciousness from which the world of names and forms arises is beyond stress because there is no division or conflict of any sort. Truth, consciousness, and bliss exist untainted. But manifestation is based on division and polarization, and as soon as polarization arises, stress inevitably exists, for the two sides of a polarity exist in dynamic tension—supporting, clashing, struggling, and dancing with one another. This creates the experiences of change, tension, conflict, and resolution.

As long as one lives in the phenomenal world, he participates in those experiences. He takes on aspects of the stress inherent in the manifest world. The stress that one experiences depends on the particular polarization

This chapter is reprinted from Dawn *magazine, Volume 5, Number 3, 1985.*

with which he identifies. The conception of chakras, or centers of consciousness, in yoga psychology offers a systematic explanation of the primary or archetypal polarizations that one must come to terms with in human life, and thus an explanation of the primary sources of stress experienced by human beings. Whereas contemporary theories emphasize the role of external factors in creating stress, such as a death in the family, a change in jobs, or a divorce, the theory being described here focuses on the way in which stress is created by one's internal processes.

A chakra is the hub of a complex network. It is a center from which thoughts, emotions, energy, and physiological responses spring. According to yoga psychology there are seven major chakras. Each of the chakras is related to a particular archetypal theme and gives birth to a distinct mode of consciousness. In each mode of consciousness, one has an experience of himself and his world that is entirely different from that which is experienced in any of the other modes. A person's concerns, his preoccupations, his energy, his "vibration," his experience of his physical body, and the nature of his relationships, emotions, thoughts, and physical and psychological disturbances are determined by the mode of consciousness that is predominant in him at any given time. These seven modes of consciousness are ordered according to an evolutionary scale, from the most primitive to the most evolved. Each mode of consciousness has a corresponding coordinate in the human body along the spinal cord. The first or most primitive chakra is found at the base of the spine; the second is at the level of the genitals; the third, near the navel; the fourth, at the level of the heart; the fifth, at the throat; the sixth, between the eyebrows; and the seventh, at the crown of the head. The endocrine glands and other major organs of the body are located in proximity to these centers and their functioning is greatly affected by the chakra to which they are proximate. All of the archetypal dramas in life and their resultant stress arise out of the polarities generated at each of these centers. When one is enmeshed in the polarity of a particular chakra, the resultant stress leads to specific psychological conflicts, symptoms, and psychosomatic disturbances related to that chakra, its mode of consciousness, and its physiological coordinates.

At the most primitive chakra, located at the base of the spine (the *muladhara* chakra), one is preoccupied with maintaining his existence, with the struggle for survival. That concern may seem to be rather remote for a person living in a so-called civilized society, but if we look at our daily newspapers we find numerous reports of war, rape, assault, and other life-threatening situations. The majority of women in our society are fearful of being raped or mugged. They are afraid to be out alone at night, to come home in the dark, or to be alone in their house, lest someone harm them. We buy bolt locks for our doors to protect us from such occurrences, and in big cities many people also have bars on their windows. When we turn on the news, we hear of further threats, such as nuclear disasters, toxic waste, and tornados. Much of our "entertainment" on television and in the movies also involves experiences of brutality, including attacks by monsters and madmen, and other life-threatening situations. One is forced to conclude that preoccupation with survival is still very much with us in the modern world.

The stress created at this chakra leads one to experience fear, anxiety, panic, and paranoia, and it leads to particular psychosomatic conditions. For example, when an animal experiences fright, it begins to defecate. That reaction is related to the fight-or-flight mechanism. If an animal is threatened with its life, it must attack or flee. The animal first empties its bowels so that it will be better able to take action. Human beings react in a similar way in situations that are perceived as threats. An athlete before a contest or a speaker or actor about to appear before an audience may, if he feels threatened, have loose bowels. That is a normal physiological response to stress generated at the first chakra. But in some people this reaction is accentuated. They unconsciously remain under the stress of this mode of consciousness and may consequently suffer from chronic colitis.

At the second chakra (*svadhishthana*), an entirely different set of concerns comes to the fore. At this chakra one becomes preoccupied with experiencing sensory pleasure of all sorts. One seeks those experiences that give pleasure and tries to avoid those that are unpleasant. All other concerns become secondary. One attempts to repeat pleasurable experiences and becomes addicted to those objects, people, and situations that have given him pleasure. He fiercely tries to hold on to them, and that creates stress and conflict, as does his avoidance of the unpleasant. In his pursuit of pleasure, he often acts in a way that is not in accord with his better judgment and his conscience. Thus he creates conflict internally and in his relationships. When one is preoccupied with pleasure, he is bound to become addicted. And when one is addicted to objects, people, or situations, he inevitably creates stress for himself. Furthermore, in his preoccupation with seeking pleasure and avoiding unpleasantness, he ignores the needs and concerns of others and creates further conflict and strife in his relationships. He treats people as objects that give him pleasure, and he becomes possessive. In seeking pleasure he creates misery for himself and others.

The person functioning from this chakra strives for the objects of pleasure and goes through all the stress involved in gaining and losing the desired objects. He becomes anxious that he may not acquire the object of his desire, and when he has it, he is fearful of losing it. Even when he does attain what he desires, his experience of pleasure is only temporary. So he strives again or seeks to extend the experience of pleasure beyond its time. Such a person is not able to flow with the moment but seeks to stop change. Stress is created by such resistance to change. If one is unable to deal with the changes that naturally occur with the passage of time, he is bound to experience stress.

One may experience a great deal of pleasure while he is eating a delicious piece of cake or indulging in any other sensory experience. But that experience lasts only for a few moments, so he must recreate that experience or look for some other if he is to remain in a pleasurable state. A person who seeks pleasure spends most of his time pursuing but has little ability to enjoy his desired object, for he has not learned how to be in the moment. Even when he has obtained the object of his pursuit, he will be so accustomed to pursuing that he will be unable to fully enjoy it. Caught in the polarity of subject and object, he is never able to become one with the object, even when it is before him, so his experience of pleasure is incomplete. He is compelled to obtain objects of pleasure, yet is unable to appreciate them when they are obtained. He lives in a state of uneasiness and unrest. This unrest compounds itself, for the more pleasurable the object he finds, the more acutely he comes to experience his inherent separation from the object. Paradoxically, the more one pursues and experiences pleasure, the more dissatisfied he becomes. As long as one lives within a subject/object framework, he is bound to make himself miserable. Pleasure never satisfies a person; it only leads to a more desperate search for pleasure. It is like an itch that increases when scratched, like a fire that increases as more fuel is poured on it. As long as one remains within this mode of functioning, he continually lives in a world of stress and strife.

The stress that results from adopting the perspective of the second chakra leads to a variety of psychological and physical disorders. In addition to the emotional, psychological, and physical imbalances that result from the craving for sensory pleasures and the addiction to pleasing objects, one can also become disturbed when desires for sensory pleasures are repressed. It was these latter disturbances that led Freud to develop his theory of neurosis. Freud traced the origin of hysterical conversion symptoms to the repression of the drive for pleasure. Subsequent theorists, including Wilhelm Reich and Alexander Lowen, have described the neurotic character as a person who denies himself pleasure and develops a rigid muscular armoring to keep pleasurable impulses from awareness. So we see that the motivation elicited at the second chakra can lead to disturbance if it is allowed expression, and also if it is denied expression. This creates a serious dilemma for the human being. If both the expression and repression of this urge lead to emotional imbalance, how can a person rid himself of disturbance? It is not possible to transcend the stress generated at this chakra and its disturbing effects as long as one remains within this mode of consciousness. The essence of this chakra is disturbance. One's desire is a disturbance, and the disturbance elicited by desire cannot be quenched either by fulfilling the desire or by repressing it. One finds relief only when he gives up desire. In other words, one must transcend the desiring mode of consciousness. This is achieved when one substitutes the perspective of a chakra which is further along on the scale of evolution.

Yoga psychology does not take a moralistic stance in arguing for either the expression or repression of the desire for sensory pleasure. It explores the various consequences that can ensue from the stress created in this mode of consciousness, and it helps one to become aware of the way in which pleasure is intertwined with suffering. In order to transcend preoccupation with pleasure in both its expressive and repressive phases, one must adopt an entirely new perspective. The attitude which may be cultivated to escape from the entrapment of this chakra is that of contentment.

In raja yoga, the royal path, contentment is cultivated as one of ten preliminary attitudes that enable a person to transform himself. In this practice, one becomes aware of the traps in running after desires and then learns to be content with what is. One learns to see the value of what is and the dis-ease in what one desires. Here contentment does not mean complacency or indifference. Rather, it is responsiveness. One learns to appreciate what is already abundantly available rather than straining after imagined sources of pleasure. In this practice, one learns that joy and happiness are already with him but are obscured as long as he is restlessly and frantically searching for pleasure outside. He realizes that disturbance occurs when one becomes attached to pleasurable experiences or when there is a blockage, a denial of the energy of this chakra. The alternative to these ways of dealing with the energy of the second chakra is to channel it upward, to use that energy in the service of more evolved chakras. This process may be compared to the process of sublimation described in psychoanalytic theory. Many of the practices of yoga are meant to transmute the energy that is expressed through this chakra.

When one moves from the second to the third chakra (*manipura*), which is located in the area of the navel, he leaves behind the preoccupations that have been described, but he experiences a new source of stress. The third chakra is that of the ego. Here one becomes preoccupied with power, control, and status. He wants to determine whether he is liked or disliked, competent or incompetent, topdog or underdog, master or slave, worthy or unworthy, a winner or loser, an insider or outsider. These are the questions that preoccupy the ego. Every person adopts both attitudes of each of these polarities, but one is conscious and the other unconscious. Consciously one may think, "I'm the greatest! I'm wonderful! I can do anything better than anyone else," but unconsciously he will be driven by a sense of inferiority. Another person will consciously feel inadequate, incompetent, and inferior, but beneath that attitude will be a hidden megalomania. These two attitudes always go together. And each person who is caught in this chakra is bound by both of them. If you really get to know the person who brags and boasts, who thinks a great deal of himself, you will realize that beneath his bravado is a frightened little child who feels unworthy, incompetent, incapable, and powerless. He is trying to block out those feelings by asserting that he is great, that he can do anything. His is a defensive reaction. And if you talk to the person who feels unworthy and inadequate, you will find that underneath his expressions of incompetence, he feels better than anybody else. He thinks that if people actually knew him, they would realize that he is really superior. These two points of view always go together, like hand and glove.

The polarization of the third chakra creates many kinds of stress and conflict. There is the obvious stress that one experiences when he feels incompetent and inadequate. There is also the stress and anxiety experienced by the seemingly competent person who repeatedly tests himself to prove his superiority. This sort of person is continually under stress as he competes with others and seeks to maintain control and power. He thinks, "Somebody else wants my job, somebody else wants to get what I have."

The ego is a provisional center of consciousness for each person. With the development of the ego, one creates artificial boundaries and an artificial self-definition. He thereby stands out from the background, which is made of all that is not identified with the ego. At the third chakra one says, "This is me." He defines himself in a particular and limited way that enables him to take responsibility for the limited territory called "I." But at the same time, the definition assumed by the ego creates a boundary. By the very fact that a person defines a territory which he calls "I," he also defines everything outside of the ego as "not I." The ego establishes a barrier or wall around oneself. One attempts to protect whatever is inside the wall and believes that everything else is foreign to him. That boundary creates the experience of loneliness, of isolation from others.

The ordinary person takes the boundary created by the ego very seriously. Instead of understanding that the ego is merely an artificial and useful construction, he identifies with the territory laid out and he thinks, "This is mine and I must protect it; whatever is outside of my territory I can manipulate and use for my benefit." But the ego is very limited in its powers, and its territory is extremely circumscribed. The world outside that cannot be controlled is vast. Therefore anyone who is functioning from the perspective of the ego has a deep sense of inadequacy. He tries to gain more power by controlling that which has been defined as outside. He tries to bolster and fortify his ego from outside. For example, he may try to manipulate others so that they will tell him, "You're attractive," "You're brilliant," and so on to help him overcome his experience of inferiority. One's sense of self-worth in this way of functioning is dependent on what others have or do not have in comparison to him. Among the emotions generated by this mode of consciousness are envy and jealousy.

When functioning from this chakra, one must constantly be on guard, protecting and bolstering his image. One is not able to relax, for he is continuously threatened with awareness of his limitations and inadequacies. There is no sense of well-being. Nor is there any feeling of unity with others, only competition. There is no real and lasting experience of success in this mode of consciousness. For every winner there must be a loser, for every insider, an outsider. One's position is always insecure: sooner or later, it is bound to change to the opposite position.

In addition to the psychological turmoil generated by this mode of consciousness, there is a host of psychosomatic disturbances. The manipura chakra is located at the solar plexus. Those who are preoccupied with the issues of this center frequently experience stomach disorders, including ulcers. Asthma is also related to imbalanced functioning of this chakra. Asthma can result when one represses the drive for self-assertiveness that is predominant at this chakra. Rather than expressing himself directly, the asthmatic keeps his emotions rigidly controlled by chronically tensing the diaphragm and chest muscles. The adrenal glands, which are located in the area of this chakra, help to "fire a person up," to arouse him so that he may assert himself. In the asthmatic the adrenal glands fail to secrete adequately. In describing the second chakra, it was noted that both absorption in pleasure-seeking and its repression created harmful consequences psychologically and physically. Likewise, the repression of the third-chakra mode of consciousness can be as harmful as overt preoccupation with competitiveness and egoism. One does not transcend competitiveness and egoism by pretending that those urges do not exist within himself. They are transcended only when one adopts an entirely new perspective of a more evolved chakra, and when assertiveness is used within the context of that more evolved perspective.

Competition and self-assertion are not in themselves negative qualities. It is one's identification with and absorption in that mode of consciousness that creates stress. The ego center enables a person to define himself and thus to take responsibility for himself in the world. Disturbances occur because people identify with their egos and with the boundaries that the ego creates. One identifies with the desire for power and control. If one is able to observe this mode of consciousness functioning within himself and to modulate its functioning, it can become useful. This occurs when one moves to the perspective of a more evolved chakra. Then one understands that the boundary drawn by the ego is merely an artificial construction to achieve a certain purpose, that the ego does not really define who and what one is. The energy and concerns of the lower chakras can be harnessed as positive forces when one does not identify himself with them, that is, when he does not lose himself in them, and when they are used in the service of more mature ways of experiencing. Then the wish to preserve one's life helps him to maintain his existence but does not lead him to become fearful or to attack others; the energy directed ordinarily toward seeking pleasure through contact with external objects is experienced in its purity as inner radiance and bliss; and the competitive and assertive urge is used to help one realize that "I" which is universal.

At the fourth chakra, the heart center (anahata), one emerges from the stress created by narrow definitions of himself. At this center he is led out of the distinction between subject and object that characterizes the first three modes of consciousness. He now begins to recognize his unity with others. He feels empathy and selfless love. He wants to give of himself and to nurture others. He is no longer preoccupied with himself but instead focuses on fulfilling the needs of others.

When consciousness evolves to this center, one emerges from the struggles, conflicts, and emotions generated by the lower three chakras. The heart center integrates one's emotional life. All the negative emotions—depression, anger, jealousy, fear, anxiety, and so on—arise out of being caught up in the lower centers of consciousness. But when we come to the heart center, that emotional energy is transformed. In the second and third chakras, one is concerned with getting: How can I get the pleasure that I want? How can I aggrandize myself? One never feels complete. He wants more and more and is never fulfilled, no matter how much he gets. There is always something more he must have. One can never really be satisfied as long as he operates from the framework of the lower chakras. Paradoxically, when one takes the perspective of the heart center and begins giving all that he is, he never experiences lack, he never feels empty. Those operating from the lower centers think, "If I give, I'll be depleted; I'll have less." But in actuality, when one takes, he can never get his fill, whereas when one gives, he experiences the abundance from which he gives and is never depleted.

Love as it is expressed at the heart center is not understood by those functioning at a lower center because love is reinterpreted in terms of that mode of consciousness. Someone functioning from the second chakra cuts a piece of chocolate cake and says, "This is delicious! I *love* this cake!" And at the third chakra one may be possessive of another person and claim that that is love. But love as it is understood from the heart chakra has nothing to do with getting anything back, any more than the sun wants anything in return for its radiance.

Although stress is greatly reduced at this center, it is not eliminated. Stress at this chakra results from one's empathy for others. One feels another's hurt, pain, and conflict. One suffers for others. Stress also occurs when one represses his loving and empathic feelings. The person who will not allow himself to experience these feelings, who chokes off such expression, may tense the muscles in his chest region as a way of denying any feeling of love or caring. As Ken Dychtwald states in his book *Bodymind,* "Tension in the area of the heart usually indicates a state of chronic over-self-protection. The individual who holds tension in this bodymind region attempts to encase his heart and heartfelt emotions with a protective wall of armor. The armor guards against hurt and attack but also locks away feelings of warmth and nourishment."[1] Exaggerated chest breathing while holding the diaphragm rigid may contribute to the armoring that takes place in this area. Symptoms that may appear as a result of conflict and tension at this chakra include bronchial conditions and heart disease. Medical researchers have found that the Type A personality, whose characteristics include competitiveness, aggressiveness, drive, striving for achievement, time urgency, and ambition, is usually prone to heart disease. Such a person functions primarily from the third chakra and does not allow his heart center to function freely and openly.

Breath awareness and yogic breathing exercises help one to release the tension in the diaphragm and chest and to breathe more completely. They make one more aware of his emotions and help him to begin the process of transforming emotions to the experience of love and compassion. The system of raja yoga also guides one in developing attitudes and behaviors that lead him from lower modes of consciousness to the mode experience characteristic of the anahata chakra. The first step in raja yoga practices consists of five preliminary practices called *yamas*. These are non-injury, non-lying, non-stealing, non-sensuality, and non-greed. As one cultivates these behaviors, he is led out of self-protective and competitive attitudes and behaviors and other preoccupations of the first three chakras. Those are replaced with behaviors based on a sense of unity and harmony with all beings. The student who follows this practice examines his relations with others each day and evaluates them to see if he is acting in accord with these principles. When he finds he is not, he replaces the undesirable behavior with that which is more harmonious. Gradually the new way of being becomes his habit.

Whereas the heart chakra is the center of humanism, of love and concern for others, the next chakra in the evolutionary process, (the *vishuddha* chakra), is where one experiences connection with that which is transcendent. Here at the throat chakra one goes further in surrendering identification with the ego and in surrendering self-pre-occupation to that which is greater than himself. The transcendent may be experienced as God in some particular form with particular qualities. One may become devoted to any representation or facet of the Lord. When one functions from the throat chakra, he experiences being loved unconditionally and being nurtured. The mystical traditions of the East and West refer to a subtle nectar, ambrosia, and to the fountain of youth—symbols of the divine nurturance experienced at this chakra. Here one feels completely loved, and taken care of. Stress does not exist when one experiences that connection. However, those mystics who have had a taste of such divine nurturance and who then go through a separation from the Beloved experience acute agony and longing to be united once again. For example, Sri Ramakrishna worshiped and had visions of the Divine Mother. "The mother began to play a teasing game of hide-and-seek with him, intensifying both his joy and his suffering. Weeping bitterly during moments of separation from Her, he would pass into a trance and then find Her standing before him smiling, talking, consoling. . . ."[2]

Unfortunately, most people are not conscious of their intimate connection with the divine. They nevertheless have an intense need to experience unconditional love and the comfort of divine nurturance, so they project that need onto other people to whom they are related, onto public figures, or onto any of the various isms. They idealize the object of their devotion rather than seeing it for what it is. One then falls in love rather than loving, or becomes a devoted follower of an idol. Sooner or later one realizes that that which he has idolized is not what he took it to be. Then he becomes disappointed, for the object he has chosen does not meet his needs. This transference of the divine into the human sphere is responsible for much of the interpersonal conflict and stress that is experienced in the world today. The majority of people are cut off from the conscious experience of divine nurturance. They are orphans, lost in the jungle of the world, where they are looking for their ideal. Their search is doomed to repeated failure until they can see through the alluring forms and avoid becoming entangled with them. In order to fulfill his longing, one must withdraw himself from incomplete representations and establish a connection with a symbol that is a genuine embodiment of the divine.

In addition to those who are lost in false representations, there are others who have closed themselves off from the experience of receiving love and nurturance. Such people may experience constriction or pain in the throat area or malfunctioning of the thyroid or parathyroid glands. Those whose need for nurturance is unfulfilled substitute a preoccupation with physical nurturance. They may turn to food or physical contact as a way of feeling nurtured. Many people deal with insecurity, anxiety, and stress by eating, for eating is associated with the acceptance, comfort, and security they experienced as an infant. That is a poor substitute for becoming aware of the universal center of nurturance that sustains all creatures of this universe. If one does not establish trust and comfort in even the physical source of nurturance, anorexia or bulimia may result.

Real nurturance, love, and acceptance are experienced when one opens himself to the universal center that sustains all beings. Devotional prayer, chanting, and self-surrender are means for attaining that awareness. If one is not inclined toward religious symbolism, there are other avenues to become aware of the universal center of nurturance. It is not necessary to believe in a religion or in a divinity in order to find satisfying symbols of the center of sustenance. One can also experience that center of unconditional love and nurturance within. By studying myths, dreams, and other expressions of the unconscious, one can gain awareness of that force that sustains all of life and become aware of the way that it functions. When one reaches such awareness, much of the stress of human life is transcended. One is no longer anxious, for he feels fully protected. There is nothing that he needs, so there is no struggle, no unfulfilled desire. This does not imply that one ceases from acting in the world. He continues to fulfill his duties but acts out of the joy and fullness of what he has received. He becomes a conduit, spreading the unconditional love that he is continually receiving.

At this stage the stresses of worldly life are left behind, but there remains a more primary source of stress to be transcended. There still exists the stress created by the awareness of two apparent existences—oneself and the center of love and nurturance. Though most people would not consider there to be any stress in such a blissful experience, from the perspective of a still more complete state of consciousness, there is still stress caused by one remaining illusory distinction. When one reaches the sixth chakra (*ajna*), the center that is located near the pineal and pituitary glands, he becomes a sage and begins to see the unity beyond even this primary polarity. The distinction between subject and object begins to dissolve. Finally when one functions from the most evolved chakra, the seventh center (*sahasrara*), located at the crown of the head, he is fully aware that there is only One, and that all that exists is a manifestation of that One that is no different from his very own being. The purpose of human existence is to reach that awareness, in which all distinctions are transcended.

When one remains in the state of unitary consciousness, there is no stress whatsoever. However, there are intermediary states of transcendent consciousness that may be experienced along the way, and these are not free from stress. If one experiences evolved modes of consciousness without following a systematic method of yoga and without guidance from one who has mastered these states, he may experience disorientation, confusion, and even mental and emotional disturbances. Stress may be particularly acute as he tries to coordinate the experiences of the higher modes of consciousness with functioning within the world of form. The stress here is of a different nature from the stress experienced by ordinary people. For instance, one may become acutely sensitive to discordant environments. Here is an example of such stress, taken from an actual journal:

> Most of yesterday was spent in the city. . . . I maintained my own center in the midst of the crowds more successfully than at any other time since the Transition. However . . . toward the end of the day my control was not so strong, and . . . I was thrown downward into the more barren levels of personal consciousness. . . .
>
> . . . I find that when this happens it begins to be dangerous and I have to struggle in order to secure simple physical safety.[3]

One may also have difficulty in helping his body adjust to the greatly enhanced energy experienced in the awakened state:

> While in the Current, I feel exhaltation and a sense of well-being that reaches well down into the outer organism, yet this does not change the fact that the Current is a powerful energy and does tax certain powers of endurance. . . . The physical body is clearly the weakest link. . . . I can suggest the feeling, if the body is thought of as something like a ten ampere fuse, while from the transformer, just beyond, there is being delivered a current on the order of one hundred amperes at a high potential. One is constantly under a

pressure to use more than ten amperes and thus strain the fuse to the point of burning out. Yet, if that fuse is burned out, correlation with this plane is broken and the expression here will remain unfinished.

Ecstatic states, experienced after placing the body in complete trance, do not involve the same problem. But in that case very little of the Inner Consciousness is likely to be carried down through the physical brain to the nervous organism, thus resulting in a corresponding limitation of outer expression.[4]

Gradually, through systematic practice, the sage learns to maintain his heightened state of consciousness while functioning in the world. This enables him to continue living in the world while guiding others in the evolution of consciousness.

The various practices of yoga are designed to help one become free from absorption in the less evolved modes of consciousness. Yogic practices bring about disidentification with those ways of thinking and being and lead one to function from the higher chakras. The practice of meditation leads one to witness the thoughts and desires that evolve from the lower chakras instead of identifying with them and acting on them. Meditation leads one to become a witness to all of the dramas created by the polarities of the lower chakras. That witnessing consciousness is free from the stress and disturbances of these chakras. It is the consciousness of the awakened seer.

Some students are taught to concentrate on one or more of the evolved chakras in order to bring their consciousness to that level. In this form of meditation, one focuses his attention in the physical location of a particular chakra. He may also visualize a particular form (*yantra*) at that center. This practice helps to bring unconscious issues at that center into consciousness so that they may be resolved. One thereby achieves a synthesis at that chakra that eventually enables him to transcend his identification with that mode of functioning.

Each of several different paths of yoga lead one to raise his consciousness to a particular chakra. For example, practicing karma yoga (the yoga of action) leads one to give up the self-preoccupations characteristic of the lower chakras and to perform his actions selflessly and lovingly. The path of *bhakti* yoga (the yoga of devotion) cultivates surrender and the experience of being in intimate contact with the divine source of love and nurturance. Jnana yoga (the yoga of direct knowledge) leads one to transcend all polarities and to realize the underlying unity of all existence. Through the sincere and steady practice of the different facets of yoga, including the science of breath, self-study, meditation, and contemplation, one transcends all of those artificial distinctions and self-created melodramas that formerly created stress and disturbance in one's life.

CHAPTER 13

Meditation, Self-Therapy, and Self-Transformation

Swami Rama

In considering the role of meditation in self-therapy, one must know with certainty what meditation means, and how meditation can be of benefit. Is meditation a complete therapy, or does one need a therapist on whom he can lean for many, many years and still not understand himself?

It is easy to adjust to the external world, but it is not so easy to understand one's own internal states because his thoughts, emotions, desires, and appetites can dissipate the mind and lead him in many different directions. Once one understands that life does not merely consist of relating to people and acquiring the objects of the world, then he will realize that life has a higher purpose: Self-realization. First of all, one should try to understand his internal states and learn to rely on his inner resources and then it is easy to adjust to the external world.

Understanding life philosophically is entirely different than understanding life in a practical way. Sometimes modern teachers say that one can understand all the problems of life if he knows the theory and practice of meditation in its full profundity. The word meditation has actually not been defined in any of the English dictionaries. According to the *Encyclopedia Britannica* the word "meditation" means "contemplation," and "contemplation" means "meditation," so this word has not really been defined. The word "meditation" is actually somewhat like "medical," meaning "to attend." To meditate, one has to learn to attend to something with full devotion and commitment. He needs to come to know himself on all dimensions and levels. When he understands this fact, then he can begin to systematically understand the whole process of the inward journey.

No therapist in the world claims to be perfect, and if therapists are not themselves perfect, then there is no chance that they can help others become perfect. At some point one will learn that he is his own therapist; he has to be. One has to be self-reliant and avoid leaning on external crutches. He needs to obtain that kind of education which is not imparted by colleges, universities, or any other external source. When one has finished examining and learning about the external world, then he wants to know the world within. He finds that the mind is a small yardstick, and that he cannot measure the whole universe with the help of that small yardstick. He becomes disappointed. When he examines the mind as it is, he comes to know that the mind alone is neither a perfect tool nor the means to attain the goal of life. An untrained mind is a foe, while a trained mind is a friend. Therefore, training the mind is very important.

In the tradition of meditation it is explained that one has to learn to go beyond the mind to a state of tranquility, equanimity, and equilibrium. Once one attains that, then he can understand the art of living in the world by remaining unaffected and can then attain the purpose of life. One needs to adjust himself to the external world and at the same time be content within. Contentment is a great virtue. If one wants to be a student of life and attain perfection, then meditation is a prime necessity of life. Meditation is a leader among all the known methods of therapy.

Many students engage in meditational therapy, and yet they are disappointed with the results. They expect too much withut following the discipline correctly. Lacking patience, modern students would often like to reap the fruits without tilling the soil and sowing the seed. But if a student wants to work consistently with himself, if he wants to know and understand his internal states and to understand himself on all levels, then meditation is a definite way to attain that.

There are three schools or approaches to growth that are very closely related. One is prayer, another is contemplation, and the third is meditation. These three distinct methods make one aware of his innermost being, the center from where consciousness flows on various degrees and grades. The purpose of these three approaches is to lead the student to that fountainhead of life and light from where consciousness flows. From childhood onward one is taught to move from one phase to another to gain knowledge. But meditation is a journey without external movement. In this journey one does not move and yet he goes forward. In meditation one has only to learn to be still physically, to have serene breath, and a calm mind.

The Body

The student of meditation should first learn to work with his body. The body is an essential instrument, but if it is not disciplined it can create a barrier on the path of attainment. Normally, a body should be healthy and free from disease. But disease can come from three sources: worry, hurry, and curry. All psychotherapies emphasize that worry and conflict within create conflict without. If one is in conflict he cannot make decisions well. If the mind is not properly guided and directed, if it is not under control, then everything is done in a disorganized and hurried manner. Behavior is not well-coordinated. If one eats too much, does not chew his food well, or eats food without nutrients, that will make him ill as well. Thus, these three—worry, hurry, and curry—are the main sources of disease and distraction for both body and mind.

To understand oneself within and without, he will have to learn to understand his inner functioning, and to accomplish that, meditation is the best method. It is a systematic approach, which tells the student to work first with his body, not because the body is something great that can transform him, or lead him to meet God or to experience samadhi. Actually, the physical body can be a great obstacle if it is not understood well. It can become a source of pain and misery, and even a little bit of pain can distract the mind. Thus if the body is not kept healthy, the mind is constantly distracted.

To be physically still, steady and also comfortable is the first requirement of meditation. The greatest strength comes from stillness and inner silence. If one learns to be still, he can learn to enjoy that stillness and peace that cannot be provided by any object in the world.

For a man, the finest and the most satisfying of all the world's objects is a relationship with a woman, and for a woman, it is a relationship with a man. But even when people have that, they are usually unsatisfied. If, however, one learns to be still, he can experience something great and profound, something that he never imagined before because he was never taught it. But, in order to accomplish that, a state of physical stillness must be developed.

Sutra I:46 of Patanjali's Yoga Sutras describes the way a student should sit for meditation, "*Sthira sukham asanam.*" *Asanam* refers to posture, *sthira* means steadiness, and *sukham* means comfortable. Thus, the posture should be steady as well as comfortable. Steadiness of posture, according to the science of meditation, means keeping the head, neck, and trunk in a straight line. If the student systematically practices this it won't take long for him to attain stillness.

One can sit comfortably on the edge of a straight-back chair, as long as the head, neck, and trunk are aligned. That is a meditative posture called *maitri* asana, the friendship posture. Many people have strange ideas about meditative postures. They think that good posture means twisting their legs and making their form elegant. Meditation has nothing to do with the upper and lower extremities except that they should be arranged so that the spinal column remains straight and comfortably aligned.

Students often ask which meditative posture they should choose, whether they should use the auspicious pose, the accomplished pose, or the easy pose. But if the spinal column is not correctly aligned, they can choose any posture they want, and it will not help. When students learn to keep the head, neck, and trunk straight, then the limbs will not disturb the posture. If students sit correctly ten minutes a day for fifteen days, they can attain significant progress.

First, one should mentally ask himself to be still and to avoid movement. Beginners will observe that the body experiences various movements because it was never disciplined. When this happens, they mistakenly think that kundalini is awakening, but actually they have not yet accomplished anything. They have not made any consistent effort, and yet they expect inner experiences. Such superficial experiences should be discarded. Physical tremors, twitching, and shaking are not healthy signs, but disturbances resulting from lack of training. Students who are not acquainted with the subject mistakenly interpret these disturbances as the symptoms of awakening kundalini. The fact is, the body has never been disciplined, so it rebels: when they want the body to be still, it moves, and these movements have nothing to do with valid inner experiences.

In the beginning, as one sits still he will observe that the gross muscles jerk. Next the muscles twitch which is the second obstacle. When the muscles twitch or when any part of the body throbs, that is not the throbbing that yoga manuals describe as a sign of progress. It is merely the release of tension.

The third obstacle to arise is shaking; the body shakes or perspires because one is straining. If one does not prepare his mind and accept the idea of meditation wholeheartedly, then he experiences mental strain, and that may cause stress leading the body to become agitated. So first the student should learn to be still and not to attend to or think about having unusual experiences. After a few days he will observe that he is able to arrest these body movements, these throbbings, twitchings, shiverings, and shakings.

BREATHING

After attaining physical stillness, one may experience discomfort in breathing. The mind is also disturbed by the unregulated breath. Breath plays an important role in life. It helps to control the mind, and if one knows how to breathe properly he can also control his emotions. For example, if one suddenly receives bad news, even though he is not physically injured the mind is affected, and he may start to cry and sob. The breath becomes shallow, and he loses all his strength. So one thought, one negative or passive emotion, can disturb the breath, affect the motion of the lungs, and upset him on all levels. Breath is like a flywheel, and if it is disturbed, the whole mechanism within is disturbed. On the other hand, if one knows how to breathe well, he can strengthen and improve himself.

Many people jog or do exercises but do not understand the relationship between breath and activity. If one coordinates the breathing with exercise, he will find it very beneficial. During exercise one should be conscious of when pauses occur in the breath. For example, suppose that one is playing tennis: when he returns to his position he should be conscious of exhaling for twice the duration of the inhalation. Learning to do this when jogging is also really a healthy exercise.

Suppose that one inhales to a count of eight—that is his normal capacity. Everyone has his or her own individual capacity, and it should be understood and then gradually expanded. If one can inhale comfortably to a count of eight, then it will not be difficult to exhale for a count of sixteen.

When one creates physical stillness in the body, rest is provided to the muscles and to the voluntary and involuntary nervous systems. By balancing the breath one establishes a balance between intake and output. Inhalation supplies oxygen to the system. The lungs are the clearinghouse for the exchange of gases. When the oxygen is consumed, it becomes carbon dioxide, which is returned to the lungs and is expelled. This is the natural and healthy cycle of breathing. These waste gases should not be retained. Proper elimination of the waste gases does not allow toxins to build up in the body, which cause many diseases.

Sometimes even though one is not suffering from any particular disease, he still does not feel quite well. This is because of the toxins that have built up in the system— because of the carbon dioxide that has been retained in the body. Thus, if one learns to exhale efficiently, it will definitely help him remain healthy.

There are many helpful breathing exercises. For example, it has been found that alternate nostril breathing, if correctly practiced, will help eliminate emotional problems and lead to emotional balance. But such special breathing exercises will not help if one does not know how to do the most basic breathing exercise: deep diaphragmatic breathing. If this is not properly practiced, one cannot expect to make much progress. This is very important; if one does not do any other exercise but learns only to do diaphragmatic breathing well, there will still be significant benefits. If one practices this exercise for five minutes, three times a day, it can be perfected in one month's time. This natural breathing pattern is everyone's birthright. When the abdomen is gently contracted, the diaphragm moves upward, pushing upon the lungs, which expels the used-up gas. When carbon dioxide is exhaled fully, more space for fresh oxygen is created.

Shallow breathing occurs because of shallow thinking, because of shallow habits such as eating too much, a lack of activity, as well as the pattern of not being accurate, exact, or direct in life. Because of their habits, people lose the natural capacity to breathe diaphragmatically, and this results in self-created suffering. No therapist can help anyone who wants to suffer; only those who work to eliminate their own self-created suffering can be helped.

It is easy to do the diaphragmatic breathing exercise. To perform it, one should lie down in *shavasana,* the corpse posture, and put a small sandbag on the abdomen. Normally for the adult twelve pounds is the recommended weight necessary to strengthen the diaphragm. Once the habit is formed, it is no longer necessary to use the sandbag. Keeping the head, neck, and trunk aligned and the lips closed, one should push in the abdomen and exhale. The inhalation should not be forced but allowed to be natural. If this is practiced three times a day, one will be a totally transformed person in a month's time, thinking differently and feeling very energetic. He will not feel lethargic in the morning.

Once this basic exercise is mastered, students can practice other exercises. But the purpose of all these exercises is to learn to regulate the motion of the lungs consciously and mentally. Normally, the involuntary nervous system is not under conscious control, but it should be.

Once one has learned the breathing exercises and has

established coordination in the breath, then he breathes properly. Proper breathing means that the breath is not shallow, jerky, or noisy, and that there are no lengthy pauses between the exhalation and inhalation. Noisy breathing is a symptom of blockage or obstruction. Long pauses in the breath means that one is high-strung and has emotional problems. Such pauses are not created when people are happy, but occur when they are experiencing some agony, problem, or insecurity. There is a brief natural pause between inhalation and exhalation, but this should not be expanded by bad breathing habits. Such a pause, if unnecessarily expanded, can be a killer; it can create coronary heart disease.

Human beings are not only physical or breathing beings. They are thinking beings too. After understanding the value of physical stillness and serene breath, then students should learn to have a calm and balanced mind.

Meditation

The mind itself never wants to meditate, because it has never been educated, cultivated, or trained to be focused or to concentrate. Gradually one has to understand and train the mind. The mind is a train of thoughts, emotions, desires, and motivations; it is a catalog of ambitions. Habit patterns are strong motivators in life, and it is not always easy to break habits. If one has formed certain bad habits, one continues to act according to them even though he does not want to. To have a habit means that one knows he should not do something, yet feels helpless. When one tries to analyze his habit patterns, he discovers that some of them have become part of his life, and some of these habits make him helpless, motivating him to do things that should not be done. He understands this pattern, but continues to repeat the same behavior again and again.

Self-transformation is possible when one becomes sincerely committed to change; then others can also be of assistance. In therapy, one person wants to change and the other person wants to help him do so, but one has to be ready for therapy in order for a therapist to help him. In self-therapy one is his own therapist, but still he has to be honest with himself and practice within his capacity.

Breathing exercises will gradually help people change their habit patterns and transform their personalities. If one is doing something he does not like and knows is not helpful, he should start doing something different. Then the mind can eliminate the old patterns and start creating new ones. Habits can be transformed by continuing one's practice regularly and faithfully.

The system of meditation is the greatest and most powerful of all therapies. Once one has learned to be still and to regulate the breathing, then he can learn to work with the mind. At first, the mind does not want to meditate because it was never trained. People do not train themselves in meditation because they unfortunately think it is something foreign or strange, but really, meditation is needed for a foundation of human life. Food nourishes the body, and many external pleasures act as simple consolations, but when one is all alone he must understand who he is, what he is, and what he wants to do. Then he learns that he has to deal with the breath and mind.

Gradually one can understand and train the mind. If one learns to be still and to breathe well, then one can attain a state of mind that is called "the joyous mind." In the technical language of yoga, this is called "the application of *sushumna*." It is the method of leading the mind to a state of joy where true meditation is possible. Sushumna application means that the breath is made to flow equally through both of the nostrils. When one understands the basic breathing exercises, then he should pay attention to the breath flowing through the nostrils. When he becomes sensitive to the flow of the breath, he will usually find that one of the nostrils is blocked. The right channel of breath is called *pingala* and the left is called *ida*. These are the heating and cooling systems in the body; the right and left channels act to balance heat and cold respectively.

Sometimes one of the nostrils flows excessively. Those whose left nostrils flow excessively are depressed, emotional, accustomed to thinking about death and negative things, feeling insecure, and crying frequently without any reason. Those whose right nostrils flow excessively tend to think constantly of doing active things, such as drinking or fantasizing about sex. So excesssive flow of either nostril is imbalanced. For this reason, a meditator knows how to balance those tendencies. There are subtle points on this subject described by the great sages for the sake of genuine students. The sages say that by focusing the mind on the bridge between the two nostrils one can bring the breath under conscious control. Unless one brings these two vehicles of inhalation and exhalation under conscious control, the mind will be controlled by unregulated breathing.

When one focuses his attention on the bridge between the nostrils, he becomes aware of the channel of breath that is flowing. Using this awareness he can change the flow of breath through the nostrils. For meditation, neither the left nor right channels should be dominant, but a natural balance should be established in which the breath is allowed to flow freely and equally through both nostrils. If one inhales and exhales equally from both, he cannot think of anything negative. The mind will find this experience delightful, because it is then undisturbed by irregularities in the breathing process, and an inexplicable state of joy occurs. Such joy has no external cause; it does not come from the love of any object. It is called love without object. When the mind attains such a state of temporary joy, called sushumna application, one can easily lead the mind into meditation.

Some days one thinks that his meditation was very

bad, and other days that it was wonderful. The reason for these fluctuations is one's breathing pattern. Breathing can be affected by one's habits regarding food, sex, or sleep. Food, sex, sleep, and the desire for self-preservation are four forces that can change the breathing behavior. The breathing pattern can be affected negatively by irregularities or by excesses in regard to food, sex, sleep, or self-preservation. Because of the urge for self-preservation people are constantly afraid, but these are useless fears that are very dangerous, for fear invites danger. A fear is something that has never been thoroughly examined. Fear is an attempt to escape, but that is not necessary. Fear is the arch enemy of human growth and must be analyzed and conquered. These four fountains of emotions can and must be regulated.

The next distraction to attend to is the mind's constant indentification with its fluctuating activities, emotions, and thoughts. When a thought occurs, one acts on it, assuming that his thoughts are always correct, but reason does not control all of one's actions—most of them are performed unconsciously. This will not happen when one learns to avoid identifying himself with the objects of the mind, because the whole problem is constant identification with the objects of the mind. That is the reason people forget their true self. The moment such a thought comes into the mind, it overwhelms the individual. Thoughts direct the mind, action, and speech—they control the entire person.

One needs to become an observer of his thinking process. Whatever comes into the mind can be objectively observed without any disturbance. But in order to do that, the mind needs a point of focus. If one is physically sick, then the navel center, or solar plexus (*manipura chakra*), is the focal point for meditation. If one is very emotional, then he can concentrate on the heart center (*anahata chakra*), the space between the breasts. If one is intellectual, and always inclined to reason or analyze, then the space between the eyebrows (*ajna chakra*) is the proper focus. If one is creatively inclined, the hollow of the throat (*vishuddha chakra*) is the concentration point. These focal points for meditation should not be chosen for oneself, however. They should be given by one's spiritual guide. Then one can focus the mind on the proper chakra or point rather than identifying with his or her thought patterns.

At first, one may have only a small amount of success; but that will increase gradually. Slowly one learns to isolate himself from his thoughts—he no longer identifies with them. Then one is in control of himself and is no longer led by random thought patterns. This principle can be illustrated by the following simile. Suppose someone is going to fetch medicine for his bedridden mother, and on the way to the pharmacy he encounters a red light. Stopping at the intersection, he may become involved with what is going by, the new faces and new cars. He may forget his purpose at this point and fail to cross the road when the light turns green. People often become similarly lost in the world and forget their aim in life. Their minds become scattered by the charms and temptations of the world, which they mistakenly value, and they forget their real purpose. Life should not be ruled by the fluctuations of the external world; one should develop some understanding of life and learn to tap the inner strength.

Learning to witness the thinking process is an essential skill. When one learns to witness something, then he can really enjoy and understand it. But when one becomes emotionally involved, identifying himself with his thoughts, he forgets his true self.

When one begins the process of self-therapy he can gradually learn to fathom all the levels within. This is very helpful and healthy, because eventually a time of transition comes when no one else can be of help. At death, one cannot completely communicate his inner experiences to anyone— not to doctors, therapists, friends, spouses, children, or other dear people. At that time, the tongue does not move; the eyes want to see, but there is a haze over all, and darkness creeps upon one and takes over. One must be realistic and prepare for that day. If he learns how to remain uninvolved with the objects of the world, then the transition from life to death will become easy.

Meditation means physical stillness, serene breath, and freedom from identification with the objects of the mind. Through meditation, one learns to understand the Self and the not-self, and to enjoy the here and now. However, meditating for five minutes a day and then being irritable the whole rest of the day is not going to help anyone. Meditation in silence should lead to meditation in action during the day. Because spiritual teachers instruct their students to meditate for five or ten minutes a day, the students expect themselves to be transformed into perfect beings. But this is not possible without meditation in action. No matter how many teachers say that students can transform themselves with meditation in stillness alone, they are misleading their students.

Five or ten minutes of meditation is very healthful provided one also commits himself to being aware of meditation in action throughout the day. One should remember the goal of remaining uninvolved and disidentified with the objects of the world, with his feelings of attraction and aversion, and with the other thought patterns in his mind. If one gets involved in these things, he becomes biased and prejudiced, and his effectiveness is lost. Therefore one should also learn to practice meditation in action.

Meditational therapy is the highest of all therapies, but some people are not prepared for it. Preparation is a necessary preliminary step to meditation, and it starts with establishing good eating habits, an adequate exercise program, and an understanding of interpersonal relationships. Thus, one can discard his obstinacy, become gentle with others, and at the same time perform his duties in life. That is how one begins the process of meditational therapy.

Contributors

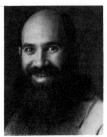 **Swami Ajaya, Ph.D.,** has practiced clinical psychology for the past eighteen years and has acted as a consultant to several mental health centers. He was educated at Wesleyan University and the University of California at Berkeley. After serving as a postdoctoral fellow at the University of Wisconsin Department of Psychiatry and teaching at the University, he traveled and studied with various sages of India, being ordained a monk by Swami Rama. Swami Ajaya is the author of *Psychotherapy East and West: A Unifying Paradigm* and *Yoga Psychology,* the coauthor of *Yoga and Psychotherapy,* and the editor of several other books.

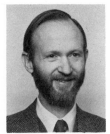 **Rudolph Ballentine, M.D.,** is president of the Himalayan International Institute of the U.S.A. After receiving his M.D. from Duke University, he studied psychology at the University of Paris (Sorbonne) and was subsequently appointed assistant clinical professor of psychiatry at Louisiana State University, New Orleans. He is presently director of the Combined Therapy Program of the Himalayan Intitute. He lectures extensively around the country and has written *Diet and Nutrition: A Holistic Approach* and coauthored *Yoga and Psychotherapy* as well as *Science of Breath: A Practical Guide.*

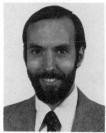

John Clarke, M.D., is chairman of the Himalayan International Institute of the U.S.A. and director of the Institute's Program in Eastern Studies and Comparative Psychology. Dr. Clarke also serves on the staff of the Institute's Combined Therapy and Research Programs. After receiving B.A. and M.D. degrees from Harvard University, he completed residency training and board certification in family practice, internal medicine, and cardiology.

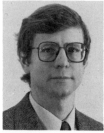

John Harvey, Ph.D., a licensed psychologist, is director of psychological services at the George T. Walter Institute of Rehabilitation Medicine, a division of Allied Services. He is a faculty member of the Program in Eastern Studies and Comparative Psychology at the Himalayan Institute. Dr. Harvey has pursued research and has published numerous articles in the areas of biofeedback, relaxation, breath, stress management, and East-West psychology. He is a contributing author of *Psychology East and West.*

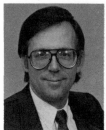

Phil Nuernberger, Ph.D., author of *Freedom from Stress: A Holistic Approach,* is on the faculty of the Himalayan Institute, where he is particularly involved in the Stress Management Program. He is a former director of biofeedback therapy at a major neurological and psychiatric clinic in the Midwest. Dr. Nuernberger serves as a consultant to several large corporations and is a contributing author to *Theory and Practice of Meditation, Psychology East and West,* and *Meditational Therapy.*

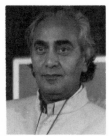

Swami Rama is founder and spiritual head of the Himalayan International Institute of Yoga Science and Philosophy. Raised in the cave monasteries of the Himalayas, he has also been formally educated in some of the most prestigious universities of both the East and West and has served as consultant to research centers such as the Menninger Foundation. He is the author of *Living with the Himalayan Masters, A Practical Guide to Holistic Health, Lectures on Yoga,* and numerous other books.

Notes

Introduction

1. *Time.* June 6, 1983, 48-54.
2. Robert S. Eliot and Dennis L. Breo, *Is It Worth Dying For?* (New York: Bantam, 1984).
3. Peter F. Nathan, "The Worksite as a Setting for Health Promotion and Positive Lifestyle Change" in *Behavioral Health,* edited by J. D. Matarazzo, S. M. Weiss, J. A. Herd, N. A. Muller, S. M. Weiss (New York: Wiley and Sons, 1984), 1063.

Chapter 1: An Overview

1. Hans Selye, *The Stress of Life* (New York: McGraw-Hill, 1976), 55.
2. Ibid., 28.
3. Mary F. Asterita, *The Physiology of Stress* (New York: Human Sciences Press, 1985), 185.
4. Ibid., 192.
5. Robert S. Eliot and Dennis L. Breo, *Is It Worth Dying For?* (New York: Bantam, 1984), 57.
6. Thomas Holmes and R. H. Rahe, "The Social Readjustment Rating Scale," *Journal of Psychosomatic Research* 11:213-218, 1967.
7. A. DeLongis, J. C. Coyne, G. Dakof, S. Folkman, and R. S. Lazarus, "Relationship of Daily Hassles, Uplifts and Major Life Events to Health Status," *Health Psychology* 1:119-136, 1982.
8. Meyer Friedman and Ray H. Rosenman, *Type A Behavior and Your Heart* (New York: Fawcett, 1974), 84.

9. John Harvey and Duncan Currey, "Patterns of Response to Stressful Tasks: A Comparison of Pain Patients, Normals and Individuals Trained in Relaxation," *Research Bulletin of the Himalayan Institute* 4 (1): 3-8, 1982.

10. Robert M. Sapolsky, "Stress and the Successful Baboon," *Psychology Today* (September 1984), 60-65.

11. Ibid., 63.

Chapter 5: The Mind and Stress

1. Hans Selye, *The Stress of Life* (New York: McGraw-Hill, 1978), 85.

2. Ibid., 451.

3. Ibid., 439.

4. George Mandler, *Mind and Body: Psychology of Emotion and Stress* (New York: W. W. Norton and Co. 1984), 124.

5. Hermann Witte, *Coping Effectively With Life* (Omaha, Nebraska: Department of Preventive and Stress Medicine, University of Nebraska Medical Center, 1985), 12.

6. Ibid., 128.

7. Bengali Baba, *The Yoga Sutras of Patanjali* (Delhi, India: Motilal Banarsidass, 1976), 31.

8. Ibid., 35.

9. Samskriti and Veda, *Hatha Yoga Manual I* (Honesdale, PA: The Himalayan Institute, 1976), 15.

10. Juan Mascaro (trans.) *The Bhagavad Gita* (Harmondsworth, England: Penguin Books, 1963), 67-68.

11. Maurice Nicoll, *Psychological Commentaries on the Teaching of Gurdjieff and Ouspensky, Vol III* (Boulder, CO: Shambala, 1984), 908-909.

12. Swami Rama, *Perennial Psychology of the Bhagavad Gita* (Honesdale, PA: The Himalayan Institute, 1985), 235.

13. Usharbudh Arya, *Yoga-Sutras of Patanjali, Volume I Samadhi-pada* (Honesdale, PA: Himalayan Institute, 1988), 91.

14. Swami Rama, *Perennial Psychology of the Bhagavad Gita* (Honesdale, PA: The Himalayan Institute, 1985), 467.

15. Usharbudh Arya, *Yoga-Sutras of Patanjali, Volume I Samadhi-pada* (Honesdale, PA: Himalayan Institute, 1988), 78.

16. Swami Satchidananda, *Integral Yoga Hatha* (New York: Holt, Rinehart and Winston, 1970), 176-177.

17. Bengali Baba, *The Yoga Sutras of Patanjali* (Delhi, India: Motilal Banarsidass, 1976, 66.

18. *The Teaching of Buddha* (Tokyo, Japan: Bukkyo Dendo Uyokai, 1978), 420.

Chapter 7: Meditation and the Quiet Mind

1. Bengali Baba, *The Yoga Sutras of Patanjali* (Delhi, India: Motilal Banarsidass, 1982), 66-67.
2. Shunryu Suzuki, *Zen Mind, Beginners Mind* (New York: Weatherhill, 1978), 79.
3. Swami Rama, *Lectures on Yoga* (Honesdale, PA: The Himalayan Institute, 1979), 145.

Chapter 9: Stress—A New Perspective

1. Hans Selye, *The Stress of Life* (New York: McGraw Hill, 1956).
2. Hans Selye, *Stress Without Distress* (Philadelphia: J. B. Lippincott Co., 1974).
3. Roger Sperry, "Mental Phenomena as Causal Determinants in Brain Function" in G. G. Globus and M. G. Savodnik, (eds.) *Consciousness and the Brain* (New York: Plenus, 1976).
4. Barbara Brown, *Supermind* (New York: Harper and Row, 1980).
5. L. Von Bertalanffy, *General Systems Theory* (New York: George Braziller, 1968).
6. Elmer Green and Alyce Green, *Beyond Biofeedback* (San Francisco: Delacorte Press, 1977).
7. Swami Rama, Rudolph Ballentine, and Swami Ajaya, *Yoga and Psychotherapy: the Evolution of Consciousness* (Honesdale, PA: Himalayan Institute, 1976).
8. Martin P. Seligman, *Helplessness* (San Francisco: W. W. Freeman and Co., 1975).
9. Lawrence L. LeShan, *You Can Fight for Your Life* (New York: M. Evans and Co., 1977).
10. Swami Rama, *Lectures on Yoga* (Honesdale, PA: Himalayan Institute, 1976).
11. Swami Shivananda, *The Science of Pranayama* (Yoga-Vedanta Forest Academy Press: Sivanandagar, Dt. Tehre-Garhwal, U.P., 1971).
12. Swami Rama, R. Ballentine and A. Hymes, *The Science of Breath* (Honesdale, PA: Himalayan Institute, 1979).
13. F. Alexander and L. J. Saul, "Respiration and Personality—A Preliminary Report: Part I. Description of the Curves," *Psychosomatic Medicine* (1940) 2(2), 110-118.

14. J. Clausen, "Respiration Movement in Normal, Neurotic and Psychotic Subjects," *Acta Psychiatrica et Neurologica* (1951), Suppl. 68, 1-74.

15. D. L. Dudley, T. H. Holmes, C. J. Martin and H. S. Ripley, "Changes in emotion with hypnotically induced emotion, pain and exercise," *Psychosomatic Medicine* (1964) 26, 1, 46-57.

16. William M. Suess, A. B. Alexander, D. D. Smith, H. W. Sweeney and R. J. Marion, "The effects of psychological stress on respiration: A preliminary study of anxiety and hyperventilation," *Psychophysiology* 17, 6, (1980): 535-540.

17. A. L. James and R. J. Barry, "Respiratory and vascular responses to simple visual stimuli in autistics, retardates and normals," *Psychophysiology* 17, 6, (1980) 541-547.

18. J. Clarke and E. Funk, "Breath coordination during exercise," *Research Bulletin of the Himalayan Institute,* 2, 4, (1980): 12-16.

19. J. Clarke, "Characterization of the resting breath pattern," *Research Bulletin of the Himalayan Institute* 1, 1, (1979): 7-9.

20. L. A. Hymes and P. Nuernberger, "Breathing patterns found in heart attack patients," *Research Bulletin of the Himalayan Institute* 2, 2, (1980): 10-12.

21. E. Funk, "Changes in Respiration with a mental task: An experimental study," *Research Bulletin of the Himalayan Institute* 3, 1, (1980): 13-16.

22. J. Harrigan, "A Component Analysis of Yoga: The Effects of Diaphragmatic Breathing and Stretching Postures on Anxiety, Mood and Somatic Behavioral Complaints," (Ph.D. Dissertation, Penn State University, 1981).

23. T. Helbick, "A proposal and preliminary literature review for the study of the effects of thoracic and diaphragmatic breathing on cardiovascular functioning," (Unpublished paper, University of Maryland, 1979).

24. P. Nuernberger, "Personality Test Scores: Effects of stress management and breath training," *Research Bulletin of the Himalayan Institute* 2, 3, (1980): 9-12.

25. A. Hymes, "Diaphragmatic breath control and post surgical care," *Research Bulletin of the Himalayan Institute* 2, 4, (1980): 9-10.

26. N. H. Azrin and R. G. Nunn, "A rapid method of eliminating stuttering by a regulated breathing approach," *Behavioral Research and Therapy* 12, (1974): 279-286.

27. D. DasGupta, "Breathing and Cardiovascular Disease," Paper presented at the 5th International Congress on Ancient and Modern Therapies: A Synthesis for Self-Awareness (1980).

28. A. Hymes, "The Pause that Kills," Paper presented at the 5th International Congress on Ancient and Modern Therapies: A Synthesis for Self-Awareness (1980).

29. A. Hymes and P. Nuernberger, "Breathing patterns found in heart attack patients," *Research Bulletin of the Himalayan Institute* 2, 2 (1980), 10-12.

30. D. DasGupta, "Breathing and Cardiovascular Disease," Paper presented at the 5th International Congress on Ancient and Modern Therapies: A Synthesis for Self-Awareness (1980).

31. A. C. Guyton, *Textbook of Medical Psychology* (Philadelphia: W. B. Saunders Co., 1971).

32. Swami Rama, R. Ballentine and A. Hymes, *The Science of Breath* (Honesdale, PA: Himalayan Institute, 1979).

33. Swami Rama, "The science of prana: basic breathing exercises." *Research Bulletin of the Himalayan Institute* 2, 4, (1980): 1-3.

34. For more detail on this subject the reader is referred to Rama, Ballentine and Hymes, *The Science of Breath.*

35. Guyton, *Textbook of Medical Physiology* (Philadelphia: W. B. Saunders Co., 1971).

36. Ibid.

37. P. Nuernberger, *Freedom From Stress: A Holistic Approach* (Honesdale, PA: Himalayan Institute, 1981), 79-80.

38. P. Nuernberger, *Freedom From Stress: A Holistic Approach* (Honesdale, PA: Himalayan Institute, 1981), 80-81.

39. C. Sagan, *The Dragons of Eden* (New York: Random House, 1977).

40. Ibid.

41. W. Penfield, *The Mystery of the Mind* (Princeton, NJ: Princeton University Press, 1975).

42. J. C. Eccles, *Facing Reality* (New York: Springer-Verlag, 1970).

43. K. H. Pribram, "Self-consciousness and intentionality" in G. E. Schwartz and D. Shapiro (eds.) *Consciousness and Self-Regulation* (New York: Plenum, 1977).

44. R. W. Sperry, "Mental phenomena as causal determinants in brain function," in G. G. Globus and M. G. Savodnik (eds.) *Consciousness and the Brain* (New York: Plenum 1976).

45. B. Brown, *Supermind* (New York: Harper and Row, 1980).

46. F. Merrell-Wolff, *The Philosophy of Consciousness Without an Object: Reflections on the Nature of Transcendental Consciousness* (New York: Julian Press, 1973).

Chapter 10: Perception and Stress

Philip G. Zimbardo and Floyd G. Ruch, *Psychology and Life* (Glenview, Illinois: Scott Foresman & Co., 1927), 163.

2. Peter M. Milner, *Physiological Psychology* (New York: Holt, Rinehart and Winston, 1970), 103.

3. W. R. Ashley, R. S. Harper, and D. L. Runyon, "The perceived size of coins in normal and hypnotically induced states," *American Journal of Psychology* 64 (1951): 564-72.

4. Swami Akhilananda, *Hindu Psychology: Its Meaning For the West* (London, England: Routledge and Kegan Paul Lt., 1960), 29.

5. Swami Hariharananda Aranya, trans. by P. N. Mukerji, *Yoga Philosophy of Patanjali* (Calcutta, India: University of Calcutta Press, 1977), 275.

6. Ibid., 275.

7. Swami Prabhavananda and Christopher Isherwood, *How to Know God: The Yoga Aphorisms of Patanjali* (New York: New American Library Inc., 1969), 119.

Chapter 11: Stress, Helplessness and Hope

1. Two overviews of the subject of learned helplessness are by M. E. P. Seligman, *Helplessness: On Depression, Development, and Death* (San Francisco: W. H. Freeman, 1975) and S. F. Maier and M. E. P. Seligman, "Learned Helplessness: Theory and Evidence," *Journal of Experimental Psychology* 105, 1, (1976).

2. J. F. Miller, *Coping with Chronic Illness: Overcoming Powerlessness* (Philadelphia: F. A. Davis, 1983).

3. Philip Nuernberger, *Freedom From Stress: A Holistic Approach* (Honesdale, PA: Himalayan Institute, 1981), 69-70.

4. J. C. Buell and R. S. Eliot, "Psychosocial and Behavioral Influences on the Pathogenesis of Acquired Cardiovascular Disease," *American Heart Journal,* 100, 5, (1980): 723-40.

5. O. C. Simonton, *Getting Well Again* (Los Angeles: J. P. Tarcher, 1978) and Lawrence LeShan, *You Can Fight For Your Life: Emotional Factors in the Causation of Cancer* (New York: M. Evans, 1977).

6. J. B. Overmier and M. E. P. Seligman, "Effects of Inescapable Shock upon Subsequent Escape and Avoidance Learning," *Journal of Comparative and Physiological Psychology* 63 (1967): 23-33.

7. S. Mineka and J. F. Kihlstrom, "Unpredictable and Uncontrollable Events: A New Perspective on Experimental Neurosis," *Journal of Abnormal Psychology,* 87, 2, (1978): 256-71.

8. Ibid., 258.

9. C. P. Richter, "On the Phenomenon of Sudden Death in Animals and Man," *Psychosomatic Medicine* 19: 191-98, 1957.

10. Seligman, *Helplessness,* 172.

11. M. A. Hofer, "Cardiac and Respiratory Function During Sudden Prolonged Immobility in Wild Rodents," *Psychosomatic Medicine* 32 (1970): 633-47.

12. J. D. Maser and G. G. Gallup, "Tonic Immobility in Chickens: Catalepsy Potentiation by Uncontrollable Shock and Alleviation by Imipramine," *Psychosomatic Medicine* 36 (1974): 199-205.

13. M. Scarf, "Goodall and Chimpanzees at Yale," *New York Times Magazine,* 18 Feb 1973. Cited in Seligman, *Helplessness,* 174-75.

14. S. F. Meier and M. Laudenslager, "Stress and Health: Exploring the Links," *Psychology Today* August, 1985.

15. E. Staub, B. Tursky, and G. Schwartz, "Self Control and Predictability: Their Effects on Reactions to Aversive Stimulation," *Journal of Personality and Social Psychology* 18 (1971): 157-62.

16. D. Glass, J. Singer, and C. Friedman, "Psychic Cost of Adaptation of Environmental Stressor," *Journal of Personality and Social Psychology* 12 (1969): 200.

17. J. Koufer and M. Seidner, "Self Control: Factors Enhancing Tolerance of Noxious Stimulation," *Journal of Personality and Social Psychology* 25 (1973): 381.

18. F. W. Thornton and P. D. Jacobs, "Learned Helplessness in Human Subjects," *Journal of Experimental Psychology* 87 (1971): 369.

19. LeShan, *You Can Fight For Your Life: Emotional Factors in the Causation of Cancer* (New York: M. Evans, 1977) 81.

20. Simonton, *Getting Well Again* (Los Angeles: J. P. Tarcher, 1978).

21. Buell and Eliot, "Psychosocial and Behavioral Influences on the Pathogenesis of Acquired Cardiovascular Disease," *American Heart Journal,* 100, 5 (1980), 730.

22. Ibid., 731.

23. W. B. Cannon, "Voodoo Death," *American Anthropologist* 44 (1942): 176.

24. R. J. W. Burrell, "The Possible Bearing of Curse Death and Other Factors in Bantu Culture on the Etiology of Myocardial Infarction," in T. N. James and J. W. Keys, eds., *The Etiology of Myocardial Infarction* (Boston: Little, Brown, 1963), 95-97.

25. Seligman, *Helplessness,* 177.

26. G. L. Engel, "Sudden and Rapid Death During Psychological Stress: Folklore or Folkwisdom?" *Annals of Internal Medicine* 74 (1971): 771-82.

27. Seligman, *Helplessness,* 183.

28. N. A. Ferrari, "Institutionalization and Attitude Change in an Aged Population: A Field Study and Dissident Theory" (Ph.D. diss., Case Western Reserve University, 1982).

29. D. R. Aleksondiowicz, "Fire and Its Aftermath on a Geriatric Ward," *Bulletin of the Menninger Clinic* 25 (1981): 23-32.

30. For a good discussion of this subject, see Swami Rama, Rudolph Ballentine, M.D., and Swami Ajaya, *Yoga and Psychotherapy: The Evolution of Consciousness* (Honesdale, PA: Himalayan Institute, 1976), 63-100.

31. A. T. Beck, A. J. Rush, B. F. Shaw, and G. Emory, *Cognitive Therapy of Depression* (New York: Guilford, 1979).

32. LeShan, *You Can Fight for Your Life,* 3.

33. Ibid., 37.

34. Simonton, *Getting Well Again,* 63.

35. Miller, *Coping With Chronic Illness,* 291.

36. Engel, "Sudden and Rapid Death."

37. Tarthung Tulku, *Skillful Means* (Oakland, Calif.: Dharma 1978), 48.

38. Miller, *Coping With Chronic Illness,* 287.

39. Viktor E. Frankl, *Man's Search for Meaning,* (Pocket Books, New York, 1963), 116-117.

40. LeShan, *You Can Fight For Your Life,* 13.

41. Miller, *Coping With Chronic Illness,* 26.

42. Beck et al., *Cognitive Therapy of Depression.*

43. Miller, *Coping With Chronic Illness,* 293.

44. LeShan, *You Can Fight For Your Life,* 145.

45. Ibid., 136-37.

46. Miller, *Coping With Chronic Illness,* 242.

47. For an excellent elaboration of this paradigm, see Swami Ajaya, *Psychotherapy East and West: A Unifying Paradigm* (Honesdale, PA: Himalayan Institute 1984).

Chapter 12: Chakras and the Origins of Stress

1. Ken Dychtwald, *Bodymind* (New York, Jove Publications, 1977), 145.

2. Swami Nikhilananda, *The Gospel of Sri Ramakrishna* (New York: Ramakrishnan-Vivekananda Center, 1970), 20.

3. Franklin Merrell-Wolff, *Pathways Through to Space* (New York: Julian Press, 1973), 140-141.

4. Ibid., 65.

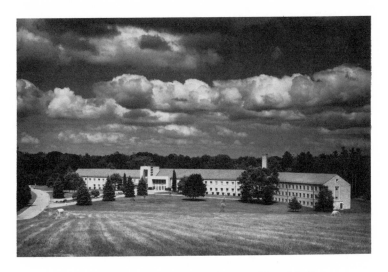

The main building of the national headquarters, Honesdale, Pa.

The Himalayan Institute

Since its establishment in 1971, the Himalayan Institute has been dedicated to helping individuals develop themselves physically, mentally, and spiritually, as well as contributing to the transformation of society. All the Institute programs—educational, therapeutic, research—emphasize holistic health, yoga, and meditation as tools to help achieve those goals. Institute programs combine the best of ancient wisdom and modern science, of Eastern teachings and Western technologies. We invite you to join with us in this ongoing process of personal growth and development.

Our beautiful national headquarters, on a wooded 400-acre campus in the Pocono Mountains of northeastern Pennsylvania, provides a peaceful, healthy setting for our seminars, classes, and training programs in the principles and practices of holistic living. Students from around the world have joined us here to attend programs in such diverse areas as biofeedback and stress reduction, hatha yoga, meditation, diet and nutrition, philosophy and metaphysics, and practical psychology for better living. We see the realization of our human potentials as a lifelong quest, leading to increased health, creativity, happiness, awareness, and improving the quality of life.

The Institute is a nonprofit organization. Your membership in the Institute helps to support its programs. Please call or write for information on becoming a member.

Institute Programs, Services, and Facilities

All Institute programs share an emphasis on conscious, holistic living and personal self-development. You may enjoy any of a number of diverse programs, including:

- Special weekend or extended seminars to teach skills and techniques for increasing your ability to be healthy and enjoy life
- Holistic health services
- Professional training for health professionals
- Meditation retreats and advanced meditation instruction
- Cooking and nutritional training
- Hatha yoga and exercise workshops
- Residential programs for self-development

The Himalayan Institute Charitable Hospital

A major aspect of the Institute's work around the world is its support of the construction and management of a modern, comprehensive hospital and holistic health facility in the mountain area of Dehra Dun, India. Outpatient facilities are already providing medical care to those in need, and mobile units have been equipped to visit outlying villages. Construction work on the main hospital building is progressing as scheduled.

We welcome financial support to help with the construction and the provision of services. We also welcome donations of medical supplies, equipment, or professional expertise. If you would like further information on the Hospital, please contact us.

Himalayan Institute Publications

Art of Joyful Living	Swami Rama
Book of Wisdom (Ishopanishad)	Swami Rama
A Call to Humanity	Swami Rama
Celestial Song/Gobind Geet	Swami Rama
Choosing a Path	Swami Rama
The Cosmic Drama: Bichitra Natak	Swami Rama
Enlightenment Without God	Swami Rama
Exercise Without Movement	Swami Rama
Freedom from the Bondage of Karma	Swami Rama
Indian Music, Volume I	Swami Rama
Inspired Thoughts of Swami Rama	Swami Rama
Japji: Meditation in Sikhism	Swami Rama
Lectures on Yoga	Swami Rama
Life Here and Hereafter	Swami Rama
Living with the Himalayan Masters	Swami Rama
Love and Family Life	Swami Rama
Love Whispers	Swami Rama
Meditation and Its Practice	Swami Rama
Nitnem	Swami Rama
Path of Fire and Light, Vol. I	Swami Rama
Path of Fire and Light, Vol. II	Swami Rama
Perennial Psychology of the Bhagavad Gita	Swami Rama
A Practical Guide to Holistic Health	Swami Rama
Sukhamani Sahib: Fountain of Eternal Joy	Swami Rama
The Valmiki Ramayana Retold in Verse	Swami Rama
The Wisdom of the Ancient Sages	Swami Rama
Creative Use of Emotion	Swami Rama, Swami Ajaya
Science of Breath	Swami Rama, Rudolph Ballentine, M.D., Alan Hymes, M.D.
Yoga and Psychotherapy	Swami Rama, Rudolph Ballentine, M.D., Swami Ajaya, Ph.D.
The Mystical Poems of Kabir	Swami Rama, Robert Regli
Yoga-sutras of Patanjali	Usharbudh Arya, D.Litt.
Superconscious Meditation	Usharbudh Arya, D.Litt.
Mantra and Meditation	Usharbudh Arya, D.Litt.
Philosophy of Hatha Yoga	Usharbudh Arya, D.Litt.
Meditation and the Art of Dying	Usharbudh Arya, D.Litt.
God	Usharbudh Arya, D.Litt.
Psychotherapy East and West	Swami Ajaya, Ph.D.
Yoga Psychology	Swami Ajaya, Ph.D.

Diet and Nutrition	Rudolph Ballentine, M.D.
Joints and Glands Exercises	Rudolph Ballentine, M.D. (ed.)
Transition to Vegetarianism	Rudolph Ballentine, M.D.
Theory and Practice of Meditation	Rudolph Ballentine, M.D. (ed.)
Freedom from Stress	Phil Nuernberger, Ph.D.
Science Studies Yoga	James Funderburk, Ph.D.
Homeopathic Remedies	Dale Buegel, M.D., Blair Lewis, P.A.-C, Dennis Chernin, M.D., M.P.H.
Hatha Yoga Manual I	Samskrti and Veda
Hatha Yoga Manual II	Samskrti and Judith Franks
Seven Systems of Indian Philosophy	Rajmani Tigunait, Ph.D.
Shakti Sadhana: Steps to Samadhi	Rajmani Tigunait, Ph.D.
The Tradition of the Himalayan Masters	Rajmani Tigunait, Ph.D.
Yoga on War and Peace	Rajmani Tigunait, Ph.D.
Sikh Gurus	K.S. Duggal
Philosophy and Faith of Sikhism	K.S. Duggal
The Quiet Mind	John Harvey, Ph.D. (ed.)
Himalayan Mountain Cookery	Martha Ballentine
The Man Who Never Died	Dr. Gopal Singh
Yogasana for Health	Yogiraj Behramji
Meditation in Christianity	Himalayan Institute
Spiritual Journal	Himalayan Institute
Blank Books	Himalayan Institute

To order or to request a free mail order catalog call or write
The Himalayan Publishers
RR 1, Box 400
Honesdale, PA 18431
Toll-free 1-800-822-4547